# MCQs in Paediatrics

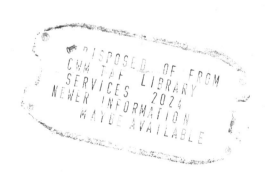

*For Churchill Livingstone:*

*Publisher:* Timothy Horne
*Project Editor:* Barbara Simmons
*Copy-editor:* Ruth Swan
*Project controller:* Nancy Arnott
*Design direction:* Erik Bigland

# MCQs in Paediatrics

With a tactical guide on how to approach clinical examinations

## Nigel Speight MA MB(Cam) BChir FRCPCH DCH

Consultant Paediatrician
Dryburn Hospital, Durham;
Associate Senior Clinical Lecturer
University of Newcastle upon Tyne

SECOND EDITION

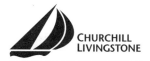
CHURCHILL
LIVINGSTONE

EDINBURGH LONDON MADRID NEW YORK PHILADELPHIA
SAN FRANCISCO SYDNEY TORONTO 1998

CHURCHILL LIVINGSTONE
A Division of Harcourt Brace and Company Limited

Churchill Livingstone, 1–3 Baxter's Place, Leith Walk,
Edinburgh EH1 3AF

© ANP Speight 1985
© Harcourt Brace and Company Limited 1998

◢◗ is a registered trademark of Harcourt Brace and
Company

First edition 1985
Second edition 1998

ISBN 0443 05777X

**British Library of Cataloguing in Publication Data**
A catalogue record for this book is available from the
British Library.

Medical knowledge is constantly changing. As
information becomes available, changes in treatment,
procedures, equipment and the use of drugs become
necessary. The author and publisher have, as far as it is
possible, taken care to ensure that the information given
in the text is accurate and up-to-date. However, readers
are strongly advised to confirm that the information,
especially with regard to drug usage, complies with
current legislation and standard of practice.

The
publisher's
policy is to use
**paper manufactured
from sustainable forests**

Produced by Addison Wesley Longman China Ltd, Hong Kong
GCC/01

# Contents

# Foreword

*by Dr John Anderson*

## How to use this book

Fifteen MCQ tests are presented; each includes 20 questions. All questions are of the multiple (independent) true/false type, with an initial stem followed by five items. Each item must be correctly identified as either 'true' or 'false'; each is independent of all the others in that question. At the end of each 'paper' the reader will find the correct answers, with a brief comment on each item. We suggest that readers should answer each test at a single sitting, allowing 45 minutes for completion. They should mark a sheet of paper T, F or D (for true, false and don't know) for each item of each question — keep individual questions separate. They should then compare their answers with those given at the end of each test. In each question one mark should be awarded for every item correctly identified as either true or false and one mark subtracted for each item wrongly identified. 'Don't know' does not influence the score. The net score for each question can then be worked out (maximum five) and when question scores are summed the total will give the percentage score for each paper.

We hope that readers will use these MCQs not only for self-assessment but also as a method of learning. It is inevitable that areas of ignorance, major or minor, will be revealed; the comments should be helpful here, but 'blind spots' should be followed up by turning to one of the standard texts so that greater knowledge can be acquired. Although an attempt has been made to achieve adequate 'balance' within individual tests, no deliberate efforts have been made to make any one test paper more difficult than another. Readers can therefore assess the progress of their learning.

## How to approach MCQs

Careful thought and the intelligent use of a sound knowledge of basic facts and principles will usually be more rewarding in the long run than plain memory work. Candidates sitting examinations can never know the level at which examiners will set the pass mark, so their sole aim must be to obtain as high a score as possible. The following hints should be helpful:

1. Read the question carefully and make sure you understand it.
2. Look at individual items one at a time, disregarding all the other

items in that question. They have nothing to do with the item you are answering.

3. Do not mark at random.

4. Do not guess. You may be lucky, but if the topic is one of which you are totally ignorant there will be an even chance that you will be wrong if you guess and you will therefore *lose* marks. Guessing is the same as saying 'heads for true and tails for false'. With a very large number of guesses the total number of marks you gain and the number you lose might even out, leaving you no worse off. But with a smaller number your 'rights' and 'wrongs' may not be equal and your chances of losing marks will be exactly the same as your chances of gaining them. This 50:50 risk is not worth taking; indicate 'don't know' if this honestly expresses your view.

5. Do not guess, but do not give in too easily. It is often possible to work out an answer that does not come to you at once by using first principles, thought and reasoning. So think carefully. If you are 'fairly certain' that you know the right answer, mark your answer sheet accordingly. In other words, be bold and play your hunches. You must try your best to make a positive response when you feel the odds are in your favour. Reasoning, deduction and thought will result in a net gain of marks. You will lose a few, but you can expect to gain more. This procedure is not guessing — it is called 'thinking'!

6. Avoid repeated review and reappraisal of your answers. Those that you were originally confident were 'absolutely correct' often look rather less convincing at a second, third or fourth perusal.

You will be able to use this book to assess the effectiveness of your reasoning power. Answer first the items about which you are completely confident and then return to the others (potential 'don't knows'). Try very hard to work out the answer and if you are reasonably confident, respond appropriately. At the end count up the number of these items on which you gained marks and the number on which you lost them. If you do not end up with a net gain, then either your reasoning ability is poor or your level of knowledge is inadequate — or both. Take appropriate action. So-called 'MCQ technique' comes down, in the end, to knowing how best to deal with items about which you are uncertain. In other words, when to give in and say 'don't know' and when to take a reasonable chance. It follows that the best way to avoid this dilemma is to reduce the chances of it arising by having a sound and comprehensive knowledge of the topic being tested.

J A

# Preface

Since the first edition of this book in 1985, there have been major advances in many areas of paediatrics and it is harder to do justice to these areas as a single author. Accordingly I have resorted to a greater degree of help from colleagues in Newcastle than in the first edition (see Acknowledgements).

The number of questions has been increased from 180 to 300 to accommodate this new material. The questions are still packaged into 20-question 'mini-exams'.

This book is aimed primarily at candidates taking the Paediatrics Part I Membership examination. It should also be of some interest to candidates for the Part I in General Medicine because of the amount of overlap between general medicine and paediatrics. This book should also be suitable for candidates for the Diploma in Child Health (DCH) and for medical students and postgraduates wishing to assess and increase their paediatric knowledge.

Section II 'How to approach clinical examinations' should be relevant to all the above groups.

I would like to endorse John Anderson's wise words in the Foreword about how to prepare oneself for MCQ examinations and how to benefit maximally from a book such as this.

Regarding overall preparations for Part I, the best advice I received on this topic was:

(i) Don't underestimate the Part I
(ii) Allow for six months of hard study.

Too many candidates enter for the Part I without having done sufficient work, simply because they are at the stage of their career where they need to pass Part I (and then Part II) to get a Specialist Registrar post.

In addition, too many candidates rely disproportionately on using MCQs as a means of study. I believe this is bad for the brain! While doing plenty of MCQs in the last couple of months is clearly important (so please do still buy this book!), these should be done *after* the acquisition of a comprehensive body of knowledge, built up systematically through extensive reading. Doing MCQs can then help (i) to assess your level of knowledge (ii) to guide you in improving your tactics and finally (iii) to help acquire 'fine points' of extra knowledge.

The stems of an MCQ should be regarded as twigs (as opposed to major branches) on the tree of knowledge.

I strongly advise candidates to try composing 10–20 MCQs themselves. They will then be better equipped tactically; for instance, they will learn to recognize the different categories of false stems (the 'plausible falsehoods' compared with the 'diametrically opposite' from the truth). They will also learn to appreciate the importance of the wording of the introduction.

Nigel Speight
1997

# Acknowledgements

Firstly, I would like to thank John Anderson for his help and guidance in the construction and refinement of MCQs to be used in the past for the Newcastle Part I course, and for his encouragement to write the first edition of this book twelve years ago.

Secondly, I would like to thank all the following colleagues in Newcastle for their help in contributing questions from their subject areas for this edition: Dr Rob Forsyth (Neurology), Dr Sally Lynch (Genetics), Dr Rod Skinner (Oncology and Haematology), Dr Mario Abinun (Immunology and Infectious Diseases), Dr Simon Hoare (Immunology and Infectious Diseases), Dr Malcolm Coulthard (Nephrology), Dr C. Harikumar (Neonatology), Dr Carol Kaplan (Child Psychiatry).

While gratefully acknowledging the above for their contributions I have applied some editorial input to the final versions and so the overall responsibility for the correctness of these questions rests with me.

The original 180 questions in the first edition have stood up to scrutiny in that I have only had one mistaken stem pointed out to me in the last 10 years. For this I would like to thank again those who helped me review questions for the first edition, who were: Hugh Bain, Simon Court, Alan Croft, Ed Eastham, David Gardner-Medwin, Edmund Hey, Bob Nelson and the late Michael Parkin.

Many of the ideas in the 'Tactical Guide to taking Clinical Examinations' derive originally from the teaching of the late Dr Maurice Pappworth, whose course for the Adult MRCP I was once fortunate enough to attend and whose department I gratefully acknowledge.

Finally, I would like to thank my secretaires Christine Burden and Denise Rewcastle for their help with typing the manuscript, which they did with their usual great efficiency and good nature.

Nigel Speight
1997

# SECTION 1

# PAPER A
## QUESTIONS

**A1** **Primary ciliary dyskinesia:**
- **A** is usually inherited as an autosomal recessive.
- **B** over 80% of cases have dextrocardia.
- **C** is associated with subfertility in the male.
- **D** can be associated with chronic serous otitis media (CSOM).
- **E** may be suspected if the 'saccharine test' is negative.

**A2** **Observation of the following occurring in relation to a headache would be compatible with a diagnosis of migraine:**
- **A** a throbbing character to the headache.
- **B** nystagmus.
- **C** symmetrical distribution.
- **D** facial pallor.
- **E** associated travel sickness.

**A3** **The following is true of X-linked agammaglobulinaemia (Bruton's disease):**
- **A** plasma cells are absent from the bone marrow.
- **B** it seldom presents before the age of 5 years.
- **C** it commonly presents with infections of the lungs and sinuses.
- **D** the underlying defect is an abnormality of the gene for B cell specific tyrosine kinase (BTK).
- **E** early replacement immunoglobulin therapy can help to prevent chronic lung damage.

**A4** **Inspiratory stridor:**
- **A** may be caused by a sternomastoid tumour.
- **B** in laryngotracheobronchitis is commonly associated with expiratory stridor.
- **C** if accompanied by a harsh cough is probably due to epiglottitis.
- **D** if chronic, barium swallow might be an appropriate investigation.
- **E** in viral croup is commonly caused by parainfluenza virus Type III.

**A5**   **Hodgkin's disease in children:**
A   occurs most commonly in the pre-school age group.
B   may present with fever and weight loss.
C   may be successfully treated with radiotherapy alone in Stage I disease.
D   is associated with cytomegalovirus infection.
E   should be investigated by a staging laparotomy and splenectomy.

**A6**   **Regarding the surface markings of the chest contents:**
A   the trachea bifurcates at the level of the 4th costal cartilages.
B   the oblique fissure starts posteriorly at the level of the spine of T4.
C   the horizontal fissure on the right is level with the junction of the sternum with the third costal cartilage.
D   the liver edge is easily palpable in 2-year-olds.
E   crepitations heard posteriorly at the level of T3 signify pathology in the upper lobe.

**A7**   **Classic features of a child with Williams syndrome include:**
A   stellate iris.
B   hypospadias.
C   hypocalcaemia.
D   hyperacusis.
E   hoarse voice.

**A8**   **Acute bronchiolitis:**
A   is caused by the respiratory syncytial virus (RSV) in over 90% of cases.
B   occurs most commonly at around the time of the first birthday.
C   if RSV is the cause then ribavirin should be used.
D   can be especially troublesome in infants with bronchopulmonary dysplasia (BPD).
E   opacities on chest X-ray are very likely to be due to bacterial superinfection.

**A9**   **In the diarrhoea-associated haemolytic uraemic syndrome (D + HUS):**
A   bloody diarrhoea is the characteristic prodrome.
B   the syndrome is caused by verotoxin, usually produced by *E.coli* 0157.
C   recurrent attacks of HUS are common.
D   if end-stage renal failure develops, HUS is likely to develop in the transplant.
E   presentation is typically with a purpuric rash over the extensor surfaces.

**A10 Regarding neonatal septicaemia:**

A  a normal C-reactive protein (CRP) is a good prognostic indicator.
B  penicillin G is the drug of choice for listeriosis.
C  intravenous gammaglobulin is an important part of treatment.
D  there is an increased risk of the neonate developing persistent pulmonary hypertension.
E  exchange transfusion may have a significant role to play in treatment.

**A11 Acute lymphoblastic leukaemia (ALL) in children:**

A  occurs more frequently in girls than in boys.
B  may present with bone pain or arthralgia.
C  is associated with a 5-year survival rate of about 70%.
D  may relapse with painless testicular swelling without evidence of haematological relapse.
E  has a better prognosis in infants than in older children.

**A12 Laboratory evidence of vertically acquired HIV infection in children includes:**

A  anti-HIV antibodies in the first 18 months of life.
B  positive viral culture.
C  hypergammaglobulinaemia.
D  low CD4 cell count for age.
E  absence of B lymphocytes in peripheral blood.

**A13 The following congenital abnormalities are deformations:**

A  talipes.
B  congenital heart defect (CHD).
C  congenital dislocation of the hip.
D  polydactyly.
E  renal agenesis.

**A14 Regarding moderate and severe learning difficulties (moderate and severe mental handicap ESN(M) and ESN(S)):**

A  the term 'moderate learning difficulties' can be used to refer to the range of IQs from 75 to 90.
B  the majority of children with 'severe learning difficulties' have a recognized cause for their handicap.
C  'moderate learning difficulties' are distributed evenly across all social classes.
D  most children with moderate learning difficulties have cerebral palsy.
E  most children with Down syndrome have IQs of 60–80%.

**A15**  **Migraine:**
  A  is commoner in females in all age groups.
  B  can cause ipsilateral lacrimation.
  C  is an unlikely diagnosis if an episode is accompanied by EEG changes.
  D  is very rare before puberty.
  E  is an unlikely diagnosis if an episode is accompanied by focal neurological signs.

**A16**  **Pre-adolescent children of mentally ill parents:**
  A  characteristically develop resilient personalities as a result of exposure to their parents' difficulties.
  B  may act in a parental role towards their parent.
  C  have a higher rate of psychiatric disturbance than control children.
  D  characteristically turn to the school for comfort and support.
  E  are statutorily required to be referred to social services for assessment of their needs.

**A17**  **Maternal conditions that may have effects in the neonatal period include:**
  A  idiopathic thrombocytopenic purpura (ITP).
  B  multiple sclerosis.
  C  diabetes mellitus.
  D  varicella zoster.
  E  Bornholm disease.

**A18**  **The following genetic disorders have a new mutation rate of above 20%:**
  A  neurofibromatosis Type I.
  B  achondroplasia.
  C  myotonic dystrophy.
  D  Huntington's chorea.
  E  Duchenne muscular dystrophy.

**A19**  **The main manifestations of vertically acquired HIV infection in children are:**
  A  Kaposi sarcoma.
  B  failure to thrive.
  C  recurrent bacterial infections.
  D  encephalopathy.
  E  opportunistic infections.

**A20**  **Definitive prenatal diagnosis is possible for the following primary immunodeficiencies (PIDs):**
  A  selective IgA deficiency.
  B  Wiskott–Aldrich syndrome.
  C  X-linked form of severe combined immunodeficiency.
  D  DiGeorge syndrome.
  E  common variable immunodeficiency.

# PAPER A
## ANSWERS

**A1**  **A**  **True**  This is a rare condition, with a prevalence of between 1:15 000 and 1:70 000. It causes bronchiectasis, sinusitis and chronic serous otitis media. It causes subfertility in both sexes. Early diagnosis is desirable to minimize lung damage, anticipate hearing problems and to facilitate early diagnosis in pre-symptomatic siblings.

**B**  **False**  50% of cases have dextrocardia (Kartagener syndrome) and 50% situs solitus. A theoretical explanation is that normal ciliary action is necessary for laevo rotation during early development, and its absence means that there is a 50:50 chance the heart will end up on the left or right.

**C**  **True**  This is due to spermatozoa having reduced or absent motility. (A different mechanism from cystic fibrosis, which is a commoner cause of the combination of bronchiectasis and male infertility.)

**D**  **True**

**E**  **True**  This test is only appropriate in adults and older children as young children cannot cooperate sufficiently. The saccharine test consists of placing a small particle of saccharine on the inferior nasal turbinate 1 cm from its anterior end. The patient must sit quietly for 60 minutes with the head bent forward and must not sniff, sneeze, cough, eat or drink during this time. In a patient with normal ciliary action, the saccharine taste will reach the tongue during this time.

The definitive investigation involves examination of samples obtained by ciliary brush biopsy.

**A2**  **A**  **True**  A throbbing character (in time with the heart beat) is well accepted as a diagnostic pointer to migraine.

**B**  **True**  Nystagmus is a well-recognized feature of basilar artery migraine.

| | | |
|---|---|---|
| **C** | **True** | Although, a *lateralized* throbbing headache with aura is accepted as 'classic migraine', a symmetrical throbbing headache with nausea would be compatible with a diagnosis of 'common migraine'. |
| **D** | **True** | Marked facial pallor (often with dark rings under the eyes) is very suggestive of migraine. |
| **E** | **True** | Travel sickness and migraine are well-recognized associations. |

**A3**

| | | |
|---|---|---|
| **A** | **True** | This condition is the commonest major immunoglobulin deficiency. There is a profound failure of B cell development, and cases present with severe bacterial infections in the first 2 years of life. |
| **B** | **False** | see (A) |
| **C** | **True** | |
| **D** | **True** | |
| **E** | **True** | |

**A4**

| | | |
|---|---|---|
| **A** | **False** | Absolute rubbish! If you ticked this you were probably tricked into thinking of a mediastinal tumour. |
| **B** | **True** | Laryngotracheobronchitis is a condition quite distinct from viral croup and epiglottitis. It is commoner in the slightly older child (1–5 years), is commonly due to secondary bacterial infection (often *Staphylococcus aureus*), and is associated with more toxaemia than viral croup. On laryngoscopy the epiglottis is normal but pus is usually seen through the vocal cords. Because obstruction is both glottic and subglottic, the stridor is usually both inspiratory and expiratory. |
| **C** | **False** | Cough is *not* a feature of epiglottitis, and is more suggestive of viral laryngitis. |
| **D** | **True** | To look for vascular rings — a rare cause but important not to miss. Compared with the commoner laryngomalacia vascular rings cause progressively increasing problems and require surgical correction. |
| **E** | **True** | |

**A5**

| | | |
|---|---|---|
| **A** | **False** | Childhood Hodgkin's disease is rare in pre-school children, being commonest in the 10–15 year age group. |

|   |   |   |   |
|---|---|---|---|
| | B | **True** | The commonest presentation is with simple lymphadenopathy. |
| | C | **True** | Stage I disease (i.e. disease limited to one group of lymph nodes only) may be treated by local radiotherapy alone. Although about 20% of patients may suffer a local recurrence, they usually respond to further treatment with chemotherapy. |
| | D | **False** | There is increasing evidence of an association between Hodgkin's disease and Epstein–Barr virus, but not cytomegalovirus. |
| | E | **False** | With the advent of increasingly accurate imaging techniques and effective chemotherapy, staging laparotomy and splenectomy is performed extremely rarely in children in the UK. |
| **A6** | A | **False** | The trachea bifurcates at the level of the 2nd costal cartilage and its junction with the manubrio-sternal joint. |
| | B | **False** | It starts at the level of the spine of T2. |
| | C | **False** | The horizontal fissure is level with the 4th costal cartilage. |
| | D | **True** | At this age the liver is $2\frac{1}{2}$ times its adult size relative to the rest of the body. |
| | E | **False** | Physical signs in this area will reflect pathology in the apical segment of the lower lobe. |
| **A7** | A | **True** | |
| | B | **False** | |
| | C | **False** | Hypercalcaemia is frequently present, and can be severe enough to cause renal damage. |
| | D | **True** | |
| | E | **True** | |
| **A8** | A | **False** | The figure is 75–80%. Other viruses that can cause bronchiolitis include influenza, parainfluenza and adenovirus. |
| | B | **False** | 90% of cases occur in the first 9 months of life. |
| | C | **False** | Ribavirin should be reserved for high risk infants, e.g. those with heart disease, BPD and immunodeficiency. |
| | D | **True** | |
| | E | **False** | In many cases, RSV alone can cause X-ray opacities, either by causing areas of collapse or actual pneumonia. |

| A9 | A | True | Virtually 100% of children present with diarrhoea and almost 70% have frank blood in it. The commonest organism responsible for diarrhoea in the UK is *E.coli* 0157 and this produces verotoxin which triggers the syndrome. Other organisms such as Shigella are commoner triggers in other parts of the world. |
|---|---|---|---|
| | B | True | See (A). |
| | C | False | D + HUS should be regarded as a rare infectious disease. A recurrence is therefore unlikely. The much less common D – HUS consists of a number of inherited syndromes in which there is a tendency to develop HUS following a trivial trigger, such as an upper respiratory tract infection. Children with this rare sub-type of HUS are therefore likely to suffer recurrences. |
| | D | False | For the same reason as in answer (C). Similarly, in D – HUS many patients *will* develop a recurrence in their transplanted kidney. |
| | E | False | Despite the characteristically low platelet count, purpuric rashes are a very rare presenting feature of D + HUS. A child with a purpuric rash over the extensor surfaces and acute renal failure is much more likely to have Henoch–Schönlein purpura. |
| A10 | A | False | The infant may have a normal CRP because he/she is too ill to mount an inflammatory response. |
| | B | False | Either ampicillin or amoxycillin is the drug of choice. |
| | C | False | IV gammaglobulin can be useful in prophylaxis of neonatal septicaemia, but has not been shown to be effective in management of an established infection. |
| | D | True | |
| | E | True | |
| A11 | A | False | ALL is more frequent in boys than girls. |
| | B | True | Bone pain can be caused by subperiostial deposits of leukaemic tissue. |
| | C | True | This figure holds for children aged between 1 and 16 years. |
| | D | True | |
| | E | False | Infants have a poorer prognosis than older children. |

**A12** **A** **False** These are not evidence of HIV infection in the first 18 months, as all infants born to HIV-positive mothers will have maternal antibodies present yet only 15% will be infected. Anti-HIV antibodies after the age of 18 months will be strongly suggestive of transmission.

**B** **True**

**C** **True**

**D** **True**

**E** **False**

**A13** **A** **True**

**B** **False** Congenital heart defects are malformations.

**C** **True**

**D** **False** Polydactyly is a malformation.

**E** **False** Renal agenesis is a malformation. The consequence of bilateral renal agenesis is oligohydramnios which can lead to deformation (Potter sequence).

**A14** **A** **False** This term is used to cover children with an IQ range of 50–70, the term 'severe learning difficulties' being reserved for children with IQs less than 50.

**B** **True** These causes include chromosome anomalies (30%), cerebral palsy (25%) and other recognized disorders such as perinatal events, meningitis and head injury. Only around 15% remain unexplained.

**C** **False** Whereas severe learning difficulties are distributed fairly evenly across the social classes, moderate learning difficulties are found disproportionately in social classes IV and V.

**D** **False**

**E** **False** The IQ of children with Down syndrome ranges from 20 to 75 with a mean of 50.

**A15** **A** **False** The sex incidence is equal before puberty and then the female predominance emerges, with 6% of boys and 14% of girls having migraine at 14 years of age.

**B** **True** Lacrimation is a feature of the migraine-related disorder of cluster headache (admittedly very rare in childhood).

**C** **False** EEG abnormalities (focal or generalized slow waves representing ischaemia) are well-recognized accompaniments of migraine.

**D   False**   If one includes abdominal migraine, the population incidence of migraine before puberty is 5–10%.

**E   False**   Focal neurological signs (hemiparesis, hemianopias, dysphasia, ophthalmoplegias, etc.) are all well-recognized features of 'complicated migraine' in both children and adults.

**A16   A   False**   While it is possible that this could apply to adolescents with previously happy childhoods, most younger children will be rendered insecure by exposure to parental deficits.

**B   True**   Having to act as a care-taker in this way is harmful to normal social and emotional development.

**C   True**

**D   False**   Children more commonly withdraw from school to look after the parent.

**E   False**   While such referral would be highly desirable in most cases, it is not statutorily required and frequently fails to occur.

**A17   A   True**   Maternal IgG antiplatelet antibodies cross the placenta and cause neonatal thrombocytopenia. There is some evidence that 'idiopathic' porencephalic cysts in older children may be the result of neonatal intracerebral haemorrhage due to undiagnosed neonatal ITP.

**B   False**

**C   True**   The worse the maternal diabetic control the more severely affected the infant. There is an increased risk of hyaline membrane disease and hypoglycaemia.

**D   True**   If the mother develops chickenpox within 5 days before or 2 days after delivery, the infant mortality is potentially as high as 5%. Accordingly the infant should receive zoster immune globulin.

**E   True**   Bornholm disease (pleurodynia, epidemic myalgia) affecting the mother in the last 2 weeks of pregnancy can lead to the infant being affected by the Coxsackie B virus and dying of myocarditis in the neonatal period.

**A18   A   True**   The figure is 50%.

**B   True**   The figure is 80%.

| | | | |
|---|---|---|---|
| | C | **False** | In myotonic dystrophy there is always an affected parent (who may be asymptomatic). |
| | D | **False** | In Huntington's chorea there is always an affected parent. |
| | E | **True** | One third of new cases are due to a new mutation. |
| **A19** | A | **False** | This is mainly found in adult patients. |
| | B | **True** | |
| | C | **True** | |
| | D | **True** | This is especially characteristic of AIDS in the paediatric age group. |
| | E | **True** | e.g. *Pneumocystis carinii*, atypical mycobacteria. |
| **A20** | A | **False** | |
| | B | **True** | The gene has been identified. |
| | C | **True** | The specific defect can be demonstrated (IL 2 receptor gamma chain deficiency). |
| | D | **True** | A deletion of a section of chromosome 22 can be demonstrated. |
| | E | **False** | This is a heterogeneous group of conditions and no genetic defect has been identified to date. |

# PAPER B
## QUESTIONS

**B1** The following is true regarding therapy for primary immunodeficiencies (PIDs):
- A gene therapy is indicated for common variable immunodeficiencies.
- B gamma interferon can be useful in chronic granulomatous disease.
- C C1 esterase inhibitor concentrate for hereditary angioedema.
- D bone marrow transplant is indicated for severe combined immunodeficiency.
- E immunoglobulin replacement is indicated for the hyper IgM syndrome.

**B2** A patient has weakness of the muscles of facial expression on the left side including those of the forehead:
- A the lesion responsible lies above the pons.
- B the left eye will roll downwards on attempted eye closure.
- C ipsilateral taste impairment may occur.
- D excess lacrimation may occur.
- E a recent history of erythema multiforme is a recognized association.

**B3** Regarding congenital malformations:
- A the offspring from first cousin matings have a congenital malformation rate of 5%.
- B the overall risk of congenital malformation in the general population is 2:1000.
- C in a family who have already produced a child with a neural tube defect, periconceptual folic acid intake is associated with a reduction in the recurrence of a neural tube defect of 20%.
- D sodium valproate intake during pregnancy is associated with an increased incidence of anencephaly.
- E lithium carbonate intake during pregnancy is associated with an increased incidence of Ebstein's anomaly.

**B4** With regard to developmental abnormalities of the respiratory tract:
- A stridor due to laryngomalacia typically worsens over the first 12 months of life.

    **B**    stridor can be caused by anomalous veins obstructing the trachea.

    **C**    stridor can be caused by bronchogenic cysts.

    **D**    glossoptosis is an important feature of the Pierre Robin anomaly.

    **E**    congenital diaphragmatic hernia is commonest on the right.

**B5**    **Corneal opacities are a recognized feature of:**

    **A**    osteogenesis imperfecta Type I.

    **B**    galactosaemia.

    **C**    Hurler syndrome.

    **D**    tuberous sclerosis.

    **E**    ataxia telangiectasia.

**B6**    **Neonatal polycythaemia:**

    **A**    occurs in small-for-dates infants as a response to placental insufficiency.

    **B**    has an increased incidence if maternal diabetes is poorly controlled.

    **C**    carries an increased risk of cerebral venous sinus thrombosis.

    **D**    is a recognized feature of congenital hypothyroidism.

    **E**    may occur as a result of feto-maternal transfusion.

**B7**    **Pulmonary haemosiderosis:**

    **A**    may be associated with glomerulonephritis.

    **B**    in its commonest form has a relatively benign prognosis.

    **C**    may be associated with a hypochromic anaemia.

    **D**    may resemble asthma in its clinical manifestations.

    **E**    chest X-ray findings may include 'miliary mottling'.

**B8**    **Conduct disorder in young adolescents:**

    **A**    carries a strong risk of antisocial personality disorder in later life.

    **B**    is mainly caused by genetic factors.

    **C**    is seldom associated with depression.

    **D**    has a good prognosis with out-patient counselling.

    **E**    has a strong association with substance abuse.

**B9**    **The following conditions are recognized causes of clubbing:**

    **A**    untreated coeliac disease.

    **B**    asthma.

    **C**    fibrosing alveolitis.

    **D**    pyogenic lung abscess.

    **E**    biliary cirrhosis.

**B10**    **Methyl phenidate (Ritalin):**

    **A**    is less effective than dexamphetamine in the treatment of attention deficit hyperactivity disorder (ADHD).

    **B**   has a half life of 12 hours.
    **C**   is not a recognized drug of abuse.
    **D**   may not be prescribed by a general practitioner.
    **E**   should not be prescribed to children less than 9 years old.

**B11**   **Pulmonary manifestations of HIV-related disease in childhood include:**
    **A**   miliary tuberculosis.
    **B**   cryptosporidial disease.
    **C**   lymphoid interstitial pneumonitis.
    **D**   *Mycobacterium avium-intracellulare* infections.
    **E**   cytomegalovirus pneumonia.

**B12**   **The following may be associated with a significant overdose of salicylates:**
    **A**   hyponatraemia.
    **B**   hypoventilation.
    **C**   metabolic acidosis.
    **D**   vertigo.
    **E**   beneficial response to desferrioxamine.

**B13**   **In the developing lung:**
    **A.**   Type I pneumocytes appear from 30 weeks' gestation.
    **B**   surfactant is produced by Type II pneumocytes.
    **C**   mucous glands are only present at 2 months' postnatal age.
    **D**   smooth muscle is not present in the bronchioles in term infants.
    **E**   the bronchi are lined by ciliated columnar epithelium.

**B14**   **Duchenne muscular dystrophy:**
    **A**   occurs more commonly in children of elderly mothers.
    **B**   is characteristically associated with a relatively low performance IQ.
    **C**   a translocation of an autosome to the Xp21 site explains why occasional affected females are reported.
    **D**   is due to mutations in the gene also responsible for causing Becker muscular dystrophy.
    **E**   is associated with increased dystrophin on immunohistochemistry of muscle biopsy material.

**B15**   **Wilms' tumour:**
    **A**   may be a cause of hypertension.
    **B**   usually presents with an abdominal mass.
    **C**   may be associated with hemihypertrophy.
    **D**   has bone marrow metastases in the majority of newly diagnosed patients.
    **E**   never occurs bilaterally at initial presentation.

**B16**   **Regarding cystic fibrosis:**
    **A**   the carrier rate in Caucasian populations is 1:100.

B    the defective gene is on chromosome 5.
C    the delta F 508 deletion is responsible for over 70% of cases in the United Kingdom.
D    female patients are usually infertile.
E    the healthy sib of a patient with cystic fibrosis has a 2 out of 3 chance of being a carrier.

**B17    Meconium aspiration pneumonia:**
A    occurs with equal frequency in term and preterm infants.
B    in infants requiring ventilation for this condition, a combination of high PEEP (positive end expiratory pressure) and rapid rates is advisable.
C    has a high risk of developing even if liquor is only thinly stained.
D    high-dose steroids are the mainstay of treatment.
E    antibiotic treatment is an important part of treatment.

**B18    The following statements concerning hereditary bleeding disorders are correct:**
A    hepatitis C virus is a common cause of liver disease in adults with severe haemophilia treated before the 1990s.
B    antenatal diagnosis of haemophilia A is possible.
C    von Willebrand disease is inherited in an autosomal recessive manner in the majority of patients.
D    children with haemophilia have a normal prothrombin time.
E    in haemophilia A, spontaneous bleeding into joints occurs when the factor VIII concentration is reduced to 20% of normal.

**B19    Regarding single gene disorders:**
A    a sibling of an affected child with any autosomal recessive disorder has a 1 in 2 chance of being a carrier.
B    tuberous sclerosis is a heterogeneous condition.
C    a sister of two boys with Duchenne muscular dystrophy has a 1 in 2 chance of being a carrier.
D    myotonic dystrophy demonstrates a phenomenon known as anticipation.
E    fragile X syndrome only occurs in boys.

**B20    Acquired immune deficiency syndrome (AIDS) in children in the UK:**
A    is most likely to be encountered in rural areas.
B    the infant of an HIV-positive mother has a 15% chance of being infected.
C    breast feeding is contraindicated.
D    most cases are due to vertical transmission from the mother.
E    affected children should be given BCG once the diagnosis is definite.

# PAPER B
## ANSWERS

**B1** **A** **False** These are relatively mild conditions, and prophylactic antibiotics are usually the mainstay of treatment, with the possible addition of immunoglobulin therapy.

**B** **True**

**C** **True**

**D** **True** The prognosis is very poor otherwise.

**E** **True** In this condition the B cells fail to switch from IgM production to IgG and IgA production. There is accordingly a deficiency of IgG which benefits from replacement therapy.

**B2** **A** **False** The patient has a *lower* motor neuron lesion of the left VIIIth cranial nerve due to a lesion of either the nucleus or the nerve itself. A lesion above the pons would be an *upper* motor neuron lesion and would spare the forehead muscles because of bilateral cortical representation. (Many people fail to appreciate that bilateral cortical representation is the *rule* rather than the *exception* for cranial nerves, the exceptions being the lower half of VII and XI.)

**B** **False** An idiopathic VIIth nerve lesion is called a Bell's palsy. Bell's phenomenon is the *upward* rolling of the eye with attempted eye closure.

**C** **True** The chorda tympani branch of VII conveys taste sensation to the anterior two thirds of the tongue.

**D** **True** Ipsilateral lacrimation may occur during the recovery phase. It is due to aberrant reinnervation and is much rarer in children than adults.

**E** **False** Lyme disease is an important cause of a facial palsy; however the rash this causes is erythema chronicum migrans, not erythema multiforme.

**B3**  **A**  **True**

  **B**  **False**  It is 2%.

  **C**  **False**  It is associated with a *70%* reduction in recurrence of neural tube defects in couples who have already had one affected child.

  **D**  **False**  It is associated with an increased incidence of spina bifida.

  **E**  **True**

**B4**  **A**  **False**  The stridor of larynogmalacia gradually improves from birth, although it may worsen during viral infections. Stridor which fails to improve or gets steadily worse should lead to investigation for other causes, e.g. aortic rings.

  **B**  **False**  Vascular rings can cause stridor, but the vessels are arteries. Their presence can be demonstrated by barium swallow, which will show indentation of the oesophagus by the vascular rings.

  **C**  **True**

  **D**  **True**  Pierre Robin syndrome consists of a midline palatal cleft, micrognathia and posterior displacement of the tongue. Glossoptosis consists of the tongue falling back and causing respiratory obstructions. Nursing in the prone position is indicated.

  **E**  **False**  The vast majority occur on the left, with bowel entering the left hemithorax and the heart shifting to the right.

**B5**  **A**  **False**  The ocular abnormality in this condition is blue sclerae.

  **B**  **False**  Untreated galactosaemia causes cataracts.

  **C**  **True**  Hurler syndrome (Type I mucopolysaccharidosis, gargoylism) has corneal clouding as an almost universal feature. This differentiates it from Hunter syndrome (Type II).

  **D**  **False**  The ocular complication of tuberous sclerosis is the presence of tubers (phakomata) of the retina.

  **E**  **False**  In this condition there are telangiectases of the conjunctiva and subsequently the face, elbows and knees.

**B6** **A** **True** Placental insufficiency causes chronic hypoxia in the fetus which, like living at high altitudes, leads to compensatory polycythaemia.

**B** **True** In poorly controlled maternal diabetes, there will be a high fetal glycosylated haemoglobin ($HbA_1C$). This is a relatively poor carrier of oxygen so again the fetus will be subjected to chronic hypoxaemia.

**C** **True** This is the rationale for performing double-volume exchange transfusion. However, simple venesection may suffice in all but the most severe cases.

**D** **True**

**E** **False** Feto-maternal transfusion will lead to anaemia in the fetus.

**B7** **A** **True** This combination is called Goodpasture syndrome and is commonest in young adult males.

**B** **False** The commonest form of haemosiderosis is the primary or idiopathic form. This is commonest in females and is associated with a chronic iron deficiency anaemia which is refractory to iron therapy. The death rate in the first 5 years from diagnosis is 50%.

**C** **True** See (B).

**D** **True** Respiratory symptoms may include cough, dyspnoea and wheeze.

**E** **True**

**B8** **A** **True**

**B** **False** Most conduct disorder is thought to be due to failings in the early environment and deficits in parenting.

**C** **False** Depression is quite common but is often masked by acting-out behaviour.

**D** **False** See (B). Such young people have very poor ability to engage with therapy.

**E** **True**

**B9** **A** **True**

**B** **False**

**C** **True** This condition does occur in childhood, albeit very rarely.

| | | | |
|---|---|---|---|
| | **D** | **True** | |
| | **E** | **True** | Patients with cystic fibrosis may have *two* reasons for having clubbing, the other of course being bronchiectasis. |

**B10** **A** **False** Both these drugs are of roughly the same efficacy in this context. Some children respond better to one drug than the other.

**B** **False** The effects of methyl phenidate wear off after 4 hours. This has practical implications for school staff, as it is in their interests to facilitate the giving of the lunch time dose!

**C** **True** Unlike dexamphetamine, methyl phenidate is not a euphoriant and has not become a drug of abuse.

**D** **False** Since 1995 it has been licensed for prescription by family doctors.

**E** **False** While fashions vary there would seem to be no rationale for restricting a therapeutic trial of such an effective drug to such a degree.

**B11** **A** **True**

**B** **False** This organism causes enteric (not pulmonary) manifestations.

**C** **True** This causes a diffuse reticulonodular shadowing on X-ray.

**D** **True**

**E** **True**

**B12** **A** **True**

**B** **False** Salicylates cause hyperventilation.

**C** **True**

**D** **True** Salicylate toxicity can cause vertigo, tinnitus and deafness.

**E** **False** Desferrioxamine is the treatment for iron poisoning or overload.

**B13** **A** **False** Both Type I and Type II pneumocytes appear by 24 weeks' gestation. Type I pneumocytes are flattened epithelial cells which constitute most of the gas exchange surface of the lung.

**B** **True** Type II pneumocytes are small cuboidal cells which are recognizable by 24 weeks and which both synthesize and store surfactant. They constitute about 15% of the total of pneumocytes.

C **False**

D **False**

E **True**

B14 A **False** There is no association with maternal age.

B **False** Affected boys characteristically show a lower *verbal* than *performance* IQ.

C **True** Duchenne and Becker muscular dystrophy are clinically-defined extremes of a spectrum of severity, all of which are due to deletions in a single gene (coding for the protein dystrophin). The gene is located at Xp21 and is inherited as an X-linked recessive. The description of occasional affected females was instrumental in localizing the gene.

D **True** As in (C).

E **False** Dystrophin is reduced or absent in affected children.

B15 A **True** About 25% of cases are hypertensive at presentation.

B **True** This mass should not be palpated repeatedly because this is thought to increase the chances of metastasis.

C **True** Known associates of Wilms' tumour include aniridia, hemihypertrophy and the Beckwith–Wiedemann syndrome.

D **False** About 20% of cases have metastatic disease at presentation, but the lungs are the commonest site for these. Bone marrow metastases are extremely rare.

E **False** About 5% of cases have bilateral tumours at presentation.

B16 A **False** At 1:25, the cystic fibrosis gene is the commonest severe autosomal recessive gene in the Caucasian population.

B **False** The defective gene is located on chromosome 7.

C **True**

D **False** Female patients have reduced fertility but successful pregnancies do occur. Male patients are usually infertile.

E **True**

**B17** **A** **False** Meconium aspiration pneumonia is a disease of term infants. Preterm infants do not produce meconium to an extent that they are at risk.

**B** **False** The biggest risk in the condition is air trapping, and therefore *low* PEEPs and slow rates are indicated.

**C** **False**

**D** **False** Steroids do not have a significant role to play. Treatment is mainly supportive although surfactant therapy may have some benefit.

**E** **False** Meconium is sterile and causes its problems by chemical irritation.

**B18** **A** **True** Unfortunately, prior to 1990 blood products were not screened for hepatitis C, and many former child patients now have chronic liver disease as a result of their treatment.

**B** **True** Haemophilia A may be diagnosed antenatally by DNA analysis of fetal blood.

**C** **False** The majority of von Willebrand disease in this country is inherited as an autosomal dominant. A small proportion (<10% in UK) have Type III von Willebrand disease which is an autosomal recessive.

**D** **True** Children with haemophilia A and B have normal prothrombin times, but raised activated partial thromboplastin times (APTT).

**E** **False** Factor VIII concentrations have to be as low as 2–10% for spontaneous joint bleeding to occur.

**B19** **A** **False** The risk is 2 out of 3. Consider the statistical model of 4 children: one is the affected child, two are carriers and one is a non-carrier. For any of the 3 non-affected children, the chances are 2 out of 3 that he/she is a carrier.

**B** **True** There are two TS genes, one lies on chromosome 9 and the other on chromosome 16.

**C** **True**

**D** **True** Anticipation in genetic disorders refers to an increasing severity of the condition with each succeeding generation.

**E** **False** Approximately one third of females who carry the fragile X gene are developmentally delayed.

**B20** **A** **False** The main risk factor for infants in the UK is being born to a mother who has been an intravenous drug user. The main centres for this are the larger cities, especially London and Edinburgh.

**B** **True**

**C** **True** This is true in developed countries, but probably untrue for developing countries, where the risks of bottle feeding are so high!

**D** **True**

**E** **False** Affected children should receive their DPT and Hib in the usual way, as these killed vaccines are safe. They should also receive pneumococcal vaccine at $1\frac{1}{2}$–2 years of age. However, BCG is contraindicated as there is a real risk of dissemination of this live virus.

# PAPER C
## QUESTIONS

**C1** **The following are true concerning the management of bacterial meningitis in childhood:**

A a serum sodium of 120 mmol/l on the third day of treatment is likely to be due to excess renal loss of sodium.

B chloramphenicol is contraindicated in the neonatal period.

C gentamicin can cross the blood–brain barrier as efficiently as sulphonamides.

D if there has been preceding antibiotic therapy and the cerebrospinal fluid reaction is totally lymphocytic, the most likely diagnosis Is tuberculous meningitis.

E cerebrospinal fluid (CSF) may be bloodstained in neonatal coliform meningitis.

**C2** **The following statements about gastroenteritis in infancy are correct:**

A the appearance of blood in the stool indicates a bacterial infection.

B secondary cow's milk protein intolerance is a recognized complication.

C the commonest identified pathogen is adenovirus.

D antibiotic therapy is indicated if a bacterial cause is implicated.

E oral rehydration fluids with sodium concentrations of 90 mmol/l are contraindicated in hyperosmolar dehydration.

**C3** **The following are characteristic features of Reye syndrome:**

A metabolic alkalosis.

B raised blood ammonia.

C cerebral oedema.

D good response to treatment with heparin.

E liver biopsy essential for management.

**C4** **The following conditions characteristically cause vesicular eruptions:**

A molluscum contagiosum.

B dermatitis herpetiformis.

C the Stevens–Johnson syndrome.

D congenital ichthyosis.

E pityriasis rosea.

**C5** The following statements are true regarding haemolytic disease of the newborn (HDN):

   **A** haemolytic disease should be suspected if jaundice is noted in the first 24 hours of life.

   **B** HDN may occur if mother is Group A Rhesus +ve and the baby is Group O Rhesus +ve.

   **C** if due to Rhesus incompatibility, the severity of the haemolysis typically increases with each affected pregnancy.

   **D** HDN due to ABO incompatibility can be detected at 36 weeks' gestation by amniocentesis.

   **E** as long as the level of unconjugated bilirubin never rises above 340 µmol/l (20 mg/100 ml) there is no danger of kernicterus.

**C6** The following are causes of polyhydramnios:

   **A** Potter syndrome (renal agenesis).

   **B** tracheo-oesophageal fistula and oesophageal atresia.

   **C** Rhesus isoimmunization.

   **D** anencephaly.

   **E** maternal diabetes.

**C7** In cyanotic congenital heart disease:

   **A** if there is cardiac failure in early infancy the most likely diagnosis is transposition of the great vessels (TGV).

   **B** there is an increased risk of cerebral venous sinus thrombosis.

   **C** clubbing is usually present at birth.

   **D** in an infant with tetralogy of Fallot, the chest X-ray characteristically shows pulmonary plethora.

   **E** tolazoline may be beneficial in cases of persistent fetal circulation.

**C8** In the long-term management of childhood asthma:

   **A** all children deserve a home-based nebulizer for the management of acute attacks.

   **B** beclomethasone by inhalation should not be prescribed continuously for more than 12 months because of the dangers of side effects.

   **C** short courses of prednisolone should only be used as in-patient therapy.

   **D** pets should be forbidden.

   **E** skin testing is of crucial importance in guiding management.

**C9** Palpable enlargement of the spleen occurs in over 75% of patients with:

   **A** Gaucher's disease.

   **B** idiopathic thrombocytopenic purpura.

   **C** hepatitis A infection.

   **D** Henoch–Schönlein purpura.

   **E** hereditary spherocytosis.

**C10**   **The following statements are correct concerning the long-term management of diabetes in childhood:**
- **A**   a child with diabetes should take less of his total calorie requirements in the form of carbohydrate than a normal child.
- **B**   the basal bolus regimen is inappropriate for children under the age of 15 years.
- **C**   if a child shows marked glycosuria yet is having frequent hypoglycaemic attacks he is probably receiving too much insulin.
- **D**   parents should not alter the dose of insulin without first seeking medical permission.
- **E**   if a teenage diabetic is planning to take vigorous exercise one afternoon, he should reduce his calorie intake at lunchtime.

**C11**   **Retinoblastoma:**
- **A**   occurs most commonly between the ages of 5 and 10 years.
- **B**   may present as a squint of recent onset.
- **C**   may cause retinal detachment.
- **D**   is relatively resistant to radiotherapy.
- **E**   has a strong familial tendency.

**C12**   **The following are characteristic features of the Wiskott–Aldrich syndrome:**
- **A**   thrombocytopenia.
- **B**   hypercalcaemia.
- **C**   eczema.
- **D**   inherited as autosomal recessive.
- **E**   increased incidence of lymphomata.

**C13**   **Minimal change glomerulonephritis:**
- **A**   is the commonest cause of nephrotic syndrome in adolescence.
- **B**   responds to prednisolone in over 90% of cases.
- **C**   is characteristically associated with highly selective proteinuria.
- **D**   is associated with hypertension in about 30% of cases.
- **E**   is characteristically associated with low serum complement levels.

**C14**   **Concerning the composition of fluids used in intravenous therapy:**
- **A**   Darrow's solution contains 36 mmol/l of potassium.
- **B**   0.18% sodium chloride and 4.3% dextrose contains 75 mmol/l of sodium.
- **C**   Hartmann's solution contains 5 mmol/l of potassium.
- **D**   1 gram of potassium chloride contains 27 mmol of potassium.
- **E**   8.4% sodium bicarbonate solution contains 1 meq/ml of sodium bicarbonate.

**C15   In the management of non-accidental injury (NAI) in England and Wales:**

A   Care Orders can only be obtained where the diagnosis of NAI is proved 'beyond all reasonable doubt'.

B   it is necessary to obtain a confession from one or other parent to confirm the diagnosis of NAI.

C   the degree of future danger is directly proportional to the severity of the initial injury.

D   a Care Order cannot be obtained for a first episode of NAI but only after a pattern of repeated injury has been established.

E   a doctor who fails to notify a case of suspected NAI is liable to prosecution by the State and a possible gaol sentence.

**C16   Anorexia nervosa:**

A   is a condition that occurs only in females.

B   may be fatal.

C   typically involves the patient having a distorted body image.

D   should ideally be managed as an out-patient with hospital admission used only as a last resort.

E   usually responds well to anabolic steroids.

**C17   The following conditions are inherited as sex-linked recessive traits:**

A   tuberous sclerosis.

B   Duchenne muscular dystrophy.

C   Ehlers–Danlos syndrome.

D   haemophilia.

E   osteogenesis imperfecta.

**C18   In the assessment and management of infantile spasms:**

A   absence of adenoma sebaceum excludes tuberous sclerosis.

B   carbamazepine is the drug of first choice.

C   there is a good prognosis for spontaneous remission of the epileptiform tendency.

D   attacks characteristically start between the ages of 3 months and 8 months.

E   treatment should only be given if the characteristic EEG findings are present.

**C19   In a case of acute paraplegia:**

A   flaccid paralysis denotes a lower motor neuron lesion.

B   traumatic lesions of the cauda equina have minimal chance of recovery.

C   joint position and vibration sense are likely to be affected if the cause is anterior spinal artery thrombosis.

D   asymmetry of leg weakness is common in poliomyelitis.

E   a possible cause is superior sagittal sinus thrombosis.

**C20** **The following statements concerning immunity are correct:**
- **A** decreased cellular immunity may lead to increased susceptibility to fungal infections.
- **B** hypogammaglobulinaemia may lead to an increased susceptibility to infections with Gram-positive cocci.
- **C** IgG levels are usually high from the age of 3 to 12 months.
- **D** decreased cellular immunity has a recognized association with hypoparathyroidism.
- **E** the immunological defect in chronic granulomatous disease is reduced efficacy of gammaglobulin.

# PAPER C
## ANSWERS

**C1**  **A**  **False**  There is no reason for excessive renal sodium loss. The most likely explanation is that the low serum sodium is secondary to inappropriate ADH secretion, which is a common complication of meningitis. This condition may aggravate cerebral oedema, and treatment consists of fluid restriction *not* the administration of sodium supplements which could be harmful.

      **B**  **False**  Chloramphenicol can be a valuable drug in neonatal meningitis due to Gram-negative organisms because of its wide spectrum and its excellent ability to enter the CSF. However, its use has largely been superseded by the newer cephalosporins. The very small risk of aplastic anaemia is insignificant when treating a condition with such a high mortality and morbidity. A far greater danger is the 'grey baby syndrome' which is a toxic dose-related effect usually due to errors in calculating or administering dosage.

      **C**  **False**  Gentamicin is an excellent bactericidal drug for systemic infections due to Gram-negative organisms. However, it crosses into the CSF relatively poorly. Because of this, some centres recommend the intrathecal and intraventricular route for administering gentamicin in neonatal meningitis.

      **D**  **False**  It would be an extremely dangerous assumption to regard such a case as due either to tuberculosis or to viral meningitis. Partially treated bacterial meningitis gives a lymphocytic CSF, and a full course of appropriate antibiotic treatment should be given in all cases with a history of previous antibiotics.

      **E**  **True**  Bloodstained CSF should not be too readily dismissed as traumatic tap or as secondary to an intraventricular haemorrhage in the neonatal period as coliform meningitis may cause bloodstained CSF. If doubt exists, it is safer to start treating for meningitis.

**C2   A   False**   Virus infections may cause bloody diarrhoea.

    **B   True**   This is quite common but distinct from the other common complication of secondary lactose intolerance. Both are usually self-limiting conditions and the treatment consists of avoidance of (i) cow's milk and (ii) lactose respectively until the condition remits.

    **C   False**   Rotavirus is the commonest identified pathogen.

    **D   False**   The only indication for antibiotic therapy is suspected septicaemia, or else undue toxaemia suggesting local invasion by, e.g. *Salmonella* or *Shigella*. The mere fact that a bacterial cause has been identified is not an indication for antibiotic therapy, as there is no evidence that such therapy is beneficial in the uncomplicated case and it may prolong the carrier state.

    **E   False**   The oral rehydration solution (ORS) recommended by the World Health Organization contains 90 mmol/l of sodium. This is a perfectly suitable fluid to use for the treatment of both hypertonic and isotonic dehydration.

**C3   A   False**   This is a rare condition of unknown aetiology in which a prodromal viral illness is followed by the acute onset of coma. Pathologically the main features are cerebral oedema with fatty degeneration of the liver. There is often a profound tendency to hypoglycaemia with metabolic acidosis, with markedly raised blood ammonia and liver enzymes. There may also be a respiratory alkalosis. Treatment is largely supportive with attempts to reduce cerebral oedema and the metabolic problems. Mortality is high. This condition appears to be reducing in incidence since a nationwide campaign to avoid salicylate usage under the age of 12 years.

    **B   True**   See (A).

    **C   True**   See (A).

    **D   False**

    **E   False**   A presumptive diagnosis made on the above features usually suffices for the purposes of management. Liver biopsy may be contraindicated as the prothrombin time is often prolonged.

**C4 A False** The lesions in molluscum contagiosum are solid. They are whitish-pink and domed or wart-like in shape. The condition is caused by a virus.

**B True** This rare condition causes large vesicular or bullous lesions especially over the lower abdomen and perineum, but also affects the face. The cause is unknown. Dapsone has been used in treatment.

**C True** Otherwise known as erythema multiforme bullosum, this condition differs from uncomplicated erythema multiforme in that the skin lesions develop vesicular centres giving the classical 'target' lesions, and also by the additional involvement of mucous membranes of the mouth, eyes and lower urogenital tract.

**D False** Ichthyosis causes a dry hyperkeratotic skin. Most forms are inherited. Lamellar ichthyosis may present in the newborn as a 'collodion baby'.

**E False** The lesions in pityriasis rosea are a combination of erythema and scaling, with the scales on each patch characteristically pointing towards the centre. The condition can be quite florid but without systemic upset, and the lesions can remain for up to 6 weeks.

**C5 A True** Physiological jaundice does not occur in the first 24 hours of life and haemolytic disease of the newborn should always be suspected in this eventuality. Since Rhesus incompatibility is usually predicted antenatally, ABO incompatibility is probably the commonest haemolytic cause of unexpected jaundice in the first 24 hours. Another important cause is infection, e.g. septicaemia. Whatever the case, jaundice in the first 24 hours should always be regarded as pathological and a cause sought.

**B False** If the baby is Group O then ABO incompatibility is impossible, as O is not an antigen and there can therefore be no antibodies to it. The commonest situation in ABO incompatibility is in fact the reverse, whereby mother is O +ve and baby is A +ve, and maternal IgG anti-A crosses the placenta and causes haemolysis.

**C   True**   Each pregnancy affected by Rhesus incompatibility can potentially worsen the prognosis for the next affected pregnancy. The mechanism is due to feto-maternal bleeding, either during pregnancy or during delivery, leading to further stimulus to the mother's immune system to produce anti-Rh antibodies. Of course, if the infant is Rh −ve this stimulus will not occur. Rhesus haemolytic disease is largely preventable if mothers are given anti-D antibody within 72 hours of delivery when the baby is found to be Rhesus +ve. This destroys the red cells of fetal origin in the mother's circulation and minimizes the antigenic stimulus.

**D   False**   HDN due to ABO incompatibility is a disease of term infants and does not significantly affect infants of 36 weeks' gestation. This is because the A and B antigens are present only in very small numbers at 36 weeks, as they are developed maximally only in the last few weeks of pregnancy. Accordingly, amniocentesis at 36 weeks is not a useful method of detecting HDN due to ABO incompatibility.

**E   False**   There is no hard and fast line below which one can safely assume that there is no danger of kernicterus. The levels of bilirubin mentioned (340 μmol/l) are customarily taken as a rough guide in term infants. However, lower levels should be used for low birth weight and preterm infants and for those with coexisting hypoxia or acidosis, as these conditions can potentiate the damage caused by bilirubin.

**C6   A   False**   In Potter syndrome there is usually oligohydramnios because of the absence of a urinary contribution to the amniotic fluid.

**B   True**   The inability of the fetus to swallow amniotic fluid in this condition leads to polyhydramnios. The infant should be checked for oesophageal atresia at birth by the attempted passage of a wide bore tube into the stomach.

**C   False**   Rhesus isoimmunization is not a cause of polyhydramnios.

**D   True**   As with tracheo-oesophageal fistula the reduced ability of the anencephalic fetus to swallow is the likely cause of the polyhydramnios.

**E   True**

**C7**  **A**  **True**

 **B**  **True**  This is due to secondary polycythaemia which leads to increased blood viscosity. Any additional illness causing dehydration will increase the likelihood of this complication.

 **C**  **False**  Clubbing takes weeks or months to develop.

 **D**  **False**  The lung fields in Fallot's tetralogy are oligaemic due to the pulmonary stenosis.

 **E**  **True**  Persistent fetal circulation is mainly a disease of term infants, and presents as cyanosis in the first few hours of life with little in the way of respiratory distress. Tolazoline, which is a pulmonary vasodilator, can be dramatically effective in this condition.

**C8**  **A**  **False**  10–15% of children have asthma and there is a wide spectrum of severity. While use of a home-based nebulizer for bronchodilator therapy may be indicated in a small minority of the most severely affected children, and in some who live far away from hospital, it is inappropriate and unnecessary in a large number of cases. There is a danger of over-reliance on a home nebulizer during severe attacks to the exclusion of hospital admission and/or steroid therapy.

 **B**  **False**  Beclomethasone has been in use for over 20 years in the UK with no serious side effects noted in long-term use.

 **C**  **False**  Short courses of prednisolone at an initial high dosage can be extremely useful in treating a child who has an exacerbation of asthma as an out-patient and thus obviating hospital admission. The danger of a life-threatening attack, e.g. on holiday or a long way from hospital, justifies giving parents an advance supply of prednisolone for emergency use. Such a policy can be life-saving and the benefits far outweigh the disadvantages.

 **D**  **False**  While occasionally a particular child may be so allergic to a cat or dog as to make continuing ownership inadvisable, the modern treatments available are so effective that in many cases the much loved pet can be preserved. Since many asthmatic children are not allergic to pets in the first place the above statement is far too strong.

**E  False**  While individual practice varies considerably most consultant paediatricians regard skin testing as of very limited importance as a guide to management. A minority perform skin tests frequently, and these are balanced by a minority who never do skin tests.

**C9  A  True**  Gaucher's disease is one of the lipidoses. There are two main forms: neuronopathic and visceral. The former presents as an acute infantile type with failure to thrive, stridor and spasticity, and life expectancy is short. The latter presents in late childhood or early adult life with pancytopenia and bone involvement, and is compatible with reasonable life expectancy. In both types hepatosplenomegaly is virtually always present.

**B  False**  Palpable splenomegaly is unusual in idiopathic thrombocytopenic purpura (ITP). Treatment of this condition may involve splenectomy in the small minority of cases which fail to remit spontaneously and are not responsive to short courses of steroids.

**C  False**  While the spleen may be palpably enlarged in hepatitis A infection, this occurs only in a minority of cases.

**D  False**  Henoch–Schönlein purpura is a condition of unknown aetiology in which purpura is due to vasculitis, not thrombocytopenia. Other features include abdominal pain and arthritis. Splenomegaly is not a feature of this condition.

**E  True**  Palpable splenomegaly is a very frequent finding in hereditary spherocytosis, and this is due to increased breakdown of the abnormal red cells in the spleen. Anaemia and jaundice are frequently just clinically detectable. The condition is familial being transmitted as an autosomal dominant. Severely affected children may need splenectomy in middle or late childhood.

**C10  A  False**  It is commonly believed that diabetics need a diet which restricts carbohydrate intake compared with that of normal children. However, there is no real rationale for this view, especially as it may lead to a compensatory increase in fat intake. The advice on carbohydrate intake should concentrate on the avoidance of excessive weight gain, the avoidance of refined carbohydrate within reason and the taking of meals and snacks in a regular and predictable way.

**B** **False** The basal bolus regimen can be well tolerated by a significant number of children under the age of 15.

**C** **True** This combination of findings is usually due to the Somogyi phenomenon, whereby excess insulin leads to hypoglycaemia, which leads to reactive hyperglycaemia probably via endogenous catecholamine release, with the possible help of growth hormone, glucagon and cortisol. Parents naturally tend to increase the insulin dosage because of the hyperglycaemia, thus aggravating the problem.

**D** **False** If parents are intelligent enough to perform blood tests and measure and inject insulin it is inappropriate to regard them as too stupid to be allowed to vary the insulin dose in response to the results of urine tests. Every effort should be made to increase the expertise and self-reliance of parents and child, as one cannot guarantee that they will always be able to get access to appropriate advice.

**E** **False** As with any subject taking vigorous exercise, increased calories are needed. To reduce the lunchtime intake is a perfect recipe for a hypoglycaemic attack on the field of play.

**C11** **A** **False** Most cases develop within the first 3 years of life.

**B** **True** If retinoblastoma arises near the macula, it will affect vision early. Loss of vision in the affected eye may lead to the appearance of a squint. At a later stage, the normal pupillary red reflux is changed to white by the tumour mass.

**C** **True** Retinoblastoma may grow between the retina and the choroid to cause retinal detachment.

**D** **False** Retinoblastoma is extremely sensitive to radiotherapy, which is fortunate in that early detection and treatment of lesions in the second eye can lead to preservation of both life and sight, even if the initially affected eye has had to be removed.

**E** **True** Each new child born to an affected family should be checked regularly for the condition over the early years of life. Almost all cases with bilateral involvement are familial, whereas most unilateral cases are non-familial.

**C12** **A** **True** The Wiskott–Aldrich syndrome consists of the following four features: (i) eczema, (ii) bloody diarrhoea, (iii) thrombocytopenia and (iv) increased susceptibility to infections. It has been difficult to explain the mechanism for the immune deficiency or to explain why these four features should coexist.

    **B** **False**

    **C** **True** See (A).

    **D** **False** This is a disease of boys and is inherited as a sex-linked recessive.

    **E** **True**

**C13** **A** **False** Minimal change glomerulonephritis usually causes the nephrotic syndrome in children from 1–5 years of age. It is a much rarer condition in adolescence, where other varieties of the nephrotic syndrome carrying a worse prognosis constitute the majority of cases.

    **B** **True** Response to steroids is extremely likely in nephrotic syndrome due to minimal change glomerulonephritis; 99% of cases may be expected to lose their proteinuria with the first course of steroids. Some will relapse off treatment and need further courses.

    **C** **True** The protein is largely albumin and IgG.

    **D** **False** Hypertension is rarely a problem in minimal change glomerulonephritis. It is more common in other causes of the nephrotic syndrome.

    **E** **False** Low complement levels are not a common feature of minimal change glomerulonephritis, and with unselective proteinuria are more suggestive of non-steroid responsive cases of nephrotic syndrome.

**C14** **A** **True** Darrow's solution was designed for the treatment of gastroenteritis, and accordingly provides both sodium (122 mmol/l) and potassium in very generous quantities. Unfortunately it is unsuitable for rapid rehydration (because of the high potassium content) and also unsuitable for maintenance therapy as it contains no calories. Half-strength Darrow's plus 2.5% dextrose is a commonly-used fluid for the second phase of rehydration, i.e. after initial resuscitation.

**B  False**  0.9% sodium chloride ('normal saline') contains 154 mmol/l (of Na and Cl) and is therefore a good fluid for extracellular fluid replacement; 0.18% sodium chloride contains one fifth the quantity of sodium, i.e. 31 mmol/l.

**C  True**  Hartmann's solution was designed as a close imitation of plasma, and contains roughly the same Na, Cl, K, Ca and $HCO_3$.

**D  False**  1 g KCl contains 13.4 mmol.

**E  True**

**C15  A  False**  The necessity to prove one's case 'beyond all reasonable doubt' is a principle of criminal justice, not civil justice. Care Orders are granted in civil not criminal courts, and a lesser degree of certainty is required, the basic principle operating being one of 'strong probability'. Failure to appreciate this fact is one of the commonest reasons why doctors refrain from making a confident diagnosis of NAI, because they imagine a 100% degree of certainty is required, which is not the case.

**B  False**  If in the course of gentle questioning one or other parent chooses to confess to having inflicted the injury this is helpful to understanding the case, and for future management, as it substantially increases the chances of successful rehabilitation. However, a confession is in no way essential for the purposes of *diagnosis*. In many cases the paediatrician has to make a firm diagnosis of NAI in the face of strong parental denial.

**C  False**  The degree of future danger can only be estimated by a thorough psychosocial evaluation of the case. 'Mild' bruising of an infant or toddler can precede a major assault that may cause death or brain damage. Severe initial injuries, e.g. fractures or subdural haematoma, may occur in a crisis in families with a good prognosis for rehabilitation.

**D  False**  Under the Children Act, a Care Order can be granted if it can be shown that the child has suffered 'significant harm' or that there is a risk of future significant harm. A pattern of repeated injury is *not* necessary for a Care Order to be granted.

**E   False**   This statement is true in the United States of America and is part of federal law. It is not true at present in the United Kingdom. In this country if a doctor's failure to report led to a child suffering repeated abuse, the doctor would theoretically be liable to a civil prosecution for negligence brought by, for example, a parent or someone acting on behalf of the child.

**C16   A   False**   While there is a very strong female preponderance in anorexia nervosa, the condition can occur in boys. The sex ratio has been reported as 10:1 in favour of females.

**B   True**   Anorexia is a relatively rare condition which is very difficult to treat, and can be fatal. One series reported contained 2 deaths out of 20 cases. Early diagnosis and specialist referral are important.

**C   True**   A distorted body image is a cardinal feature of anorexia nervosa, and serves to differentiate it from organic conditions in which the patient is anorectic but agrees that he/she is too thin. The patient with anorexia nervosa persists in regarding herself as too fat even when emaciated to the point of death.

**D   False**   Both the aetiology and therefore the management of anorexia nervosa are the subject of much controversy, in which there are two main schools of thought. The psychodynamic school of thought favours a psychotherapeutic approach, as opposed to the behaviouralists who favour an approach based on withdrawal of privileges with their return as a reward for eating. However, both sides recognize the severity of the condition and tend to favour *early* admission to hospital.

**E   False**   Various drugs have been used in attempts to treat anorexia nervosa, including chlorpromazine and tricyclic antidepressants. None is very effective and there is no evidence that anabolic steroids have a significant beneficial effect.

**C17   A   False**   Tuberous sclerosis (adenoma sebaceum) is inherited as an autosomal dominant, as is von Recklinghausen's disease, another neurodermatosis with which it shares some common features.

**B** **True** Duchenne muscular dystrophy is characteristically inherited as a sex-linked recessive, although 10% of cases are inherited as an autosomal recessive. The tragic nature of this disease renders full family studies and genetic counselling essential as early as possible. If female family members have moderately raised serum creatine kinase they are carriers, but a normal level can still be compatible with carrier status.

**C** **False** Ehlers–Danlos syndrome is inherited as an autosomal dominant. Its main features are cutaneous hyperelasticity and hyperextensible joints with fragile skin and blood vessels leading to an abnormal bleeding tendency.

**D** **True** Classic haemophilia is inherited as a sex-linked recessive, i.e. it affects males and is carried by asymptomatic females. Female carriers may be detected and genetic counselling is indicated.

**E** **False** Osteogenesis imperfecta is usually due to an autosomal dominant occurring as a sporadic mutation. A minority of cases are probably due to autosomal recessive inheritance.

**C18** **A** **False** Infantile spasms are a common presenting feature of infants who have suffered perinatal brain injury or who have a degenerative brain condition. Infants with tuberous sclerosis frequently present in this way, and at an age prior to the development of adenoma sebaceum.

**B** **False** Infantile spasms tend to be relatively resistant to the anticonvulsants used for grand mal epilepsy. In the past steroids have been the drugs of first choice, possibly combined with nitrazepam. Vigabatrin has recently been shown to be very effective in this condition and may become the drug of first choice.

**C** **False** See (A). Infants presenting in this way frequently go on to suffer intractable grand mal epilepsy often with associated mental retardation.

**D** **True** Below the age of 6 months the brain is relatively resistant to epileptiform stimuli, and infantile spasms are best regarded as the way the brain responds at this age to stimuli that would at a later age produce a grand mal convulsion.

**E** **False** While many cases will show the classic EEG changes of hypsarrhythmia a minority will not. All should be treated empirically, see (B), and a search made for degenerative brain conditions or a metabolic problem affecting cerebral function.

**C19** **A** **False** While lower motor neuron lesions do typically cause flaccidity, so do upper motor neuron lesions in the acute stage. Spasticity may take weeks or months to develop in an acute upper motor neuron paraplegia.

**B** **False** The cauda equina consists of peripheral nerves which, like all peripheral nerves, are capable of regeneration following traumatic insults. This contrasts with spinal cord lesions in which far less recovery is possible.

**C** **False** The anterior spinal artery supplies the anterior two thirds of the spinal cord. Accordingly, an anterior spinal artery thrombosis will cause a dense paraplegia with spinothalamic sensory loss, but good preservation of joint position sense and vibration, which are spared because of their position in the relatively unaffected posterior columns. This kind of sensory loss is known as 'dissociated anaesthesia'.

**D** **True** In poliomyelitis, the involvement of anterior horn cells in cervical and lumbar segments is essentially patchy, and therefore asymmetry of leg weakness in a case of polio is quite likely.

**E** **True** The area of each motor cortex which supplies the leg is at the top of the prefrontal gyrus close to the sagittal sinus. Traumatic, vascular or neoplastic lesions in this area can therefore affect both the cortical areas supplying the legs and cause a spastic paraplegia. Possible vascular causes include a septic thrombophlebitis of the sagittal sinus, or a non-septic thrombosis in, for example, severe dehydration or secondary to polycythaemia in cyanotic congenital heart disease.

**C20** **A** **True** Cellular immunity is also important in virus infections and graft rejection, and some bacterial infections such as tuberculosis.

**B** **True** These infections are the main problem in primary hypogammaglobulinaemia, which may or may not be inherited as a sex-linked recessive. Infections begin to occur with increasing frequency in the second half of the first year of life when the passive protection afforded by maternal gammaglobulin wears off.

**C** **False** There is a physiological trough in IgG levels over this period, due to the waning of maternal IgG and a delay in the production of the infant's own IgG, presumably due to lack of stimulus.

**D** **True** Both hypoparathyroidism and decreased cellular immunity are features of the branchial arch syndrome (DiGeorge syndrome). Both the parathyroids and the thymus arise from the 3rd–4th branchial arch, thus explaining this association. Congenital heart disease may be associated for the same reason. Infants may present with tetany in early life, followed by infections and lymphopenia. The gene abnormality causing this group of conditions has been localized on chromosome 22.

**E** **False** In this rare condition, which is probably inherited as a sex-linked recessive, the main defect is a failure of polymorphs to kill bacteria and fungi after phagocytosis due to an intracellular enzyme defect. The organisms continue to multiply slowly, causing granulomata in lymphoid tissue. Infants present with chronic otitis media, intractable oropharyngeal candidiasis and pulmonary and gastrointestinal infections.

# PAPER D
## QUESTIONS

**D1**   **Brain tumours in children:**
   **A**   do not present with symptoms or signs of raised intracranial pressure due to the distensibility of the skull.
   **B**   occur more commonly in supratentorial than in infratentorial locations.
   **C**   may present with deteriorating school performance.
   **D**   are metastatic from extracranial tumours in about 25% of cases.
   **E**   do not require treatment if the histology is benign.

**D2**   **Regarding genetic tests:**
   **A**   the polymerase chain reaction (PCR) is a method of amplifying short segments of DNA for genetic analysis.
   **B**   the commonest mutation in the cystic fibrosis gene in British Caucasians is a three base pair deletion known as delta F 508.
   **C**   fragile X syndrome, myotonic dystrophy and Huntington's chorea share the same mutational mechanism.
   **D**   spinal muscular atrophy Types I and II are due to different mutations in the same gene.
   **E**   a DNA fingerprinting test will show that monozygotic twins share 80% of their genes in common.

**D3**   **The following statements are true of cystinosis:**
   **A**   the plasma potassium, bicarbonate and phosphate levels are characteristically high.
   **B**   presentation is usually with anorexia, polyuria and polydipsia under the age of two.
   **C**   rickets is an early feature.
   **D**   the diagnosis can be made from a bone marrow aspirate.
   **E**   diabetes mellitus and hypothyroidism may be late features.

**D4**   **The following are true regarding cystic fibrosis:**
   **A**   Addison's disease may give a false positive sweat test.
   **B**   calcium supplements would be appropriate for a visit to tropical Africa to prevent night cramps.

   **C**   allergic pulmonary aspergillosis is associated with a polyclonal gammopathy.
   **D**   a sweat sodium of 60 mmol/l is diagnostic of cystic fibrosis.
   **E**   oral amiloride has a clinically useful role in reducing sputum viscosity.

**D5**   **A 9-year-old child has a first, single, generalized tonic-clonic seizure:**
   **A**   the risk of a second seizure is approximately 80%.
   **B**   the child should be cautioned against cycling in traffic.
   **C**   a CT scan should be performed.
   **D**   an EEG may show generalized 3 Hz spike and wave activity upon hyperventilation.
   **E**   partial seizures around the mouth could be helpful diagnostically.

**D6**   **In the psychological development of children:**
   **A**   infant temperament bears little relationship to personality in later childhood.
   **B**   infant–mother attachment occurs maximally in the first few days of life.
   **C**   the latency period refers to the approximate age range from 5 to 12 years.
   **D**   in general one would expect a child of 2 years of age to withstand a one week separation from its mother better than an infant of 3 months of age.
   **E**   basic trust versus mistrust is the first of the 'Eriksonian' stages to be negotiated.

**D7**   **Recognized features of sarcoidosis in children include:**
   **A**   conjunctivitis.
   **B**   erythema nodosum.
   **C**   facial palsy.
   **D**   parotitis.
   **E**   diabetes insipidus.

**D8**   **Regarding pertussis:**
   **A**   maternal immunity does not have a significant protective effect in the first 3 months of life.
   **B**   diagnosis is essentially clinical.
   **C**   should not be diagnosed in the absence of a whoop.
   **D**   should only be notified if cultures are positive for *B. pertussis*.
   **E**   characteristically lasts for 6 weeks.

**D9**   **Attention deficit hyperactivity disorder (ADHD):**
   **A**   has an incidence in the childhood population of between 1 and 5 per 1000.
   **B**   remits spontaneously in adolescence.

C   has a recognized association with specific learning difficulties.
D   has a higher incidence in social classes I and II.
E   includes impulsivity as one of its cardinal features.

**D10   In acute severe asthma:**
A   pulsus paradoxus reflects impending heart failure.
B   face mask oxygen should not exceed 40%.
C   intravenous hydrocortisone is best administered as a continuous infusion.
D   elective ventilation should be instituted if the $Pco_2$ rises above 8 kPa.
E   if ventilation is required, a rapid rate (> 60/min) is desirable.

**D11   Polyhydramnios:**
A   is defined as an amniotic fluid volume of more than 500 ml.
B   occurs with increased frequency in diabetic pregnancies.
C   is associated with renal agenesis.
D   is associated with tracheo-oesophageal fistula.
E   is associated with an increased risk of premature labour.

**D12   The following conditions are caused by an abnormality of haemoglobin synthesis:**
A   beta thalassaemia.
B   congenital spherocytosis.
C   pyruvate kinase deficiency.
D   haemophilia A.
E   sickle cell disease.

**D13   Regarding childhood asthma:**
A   $\beta_2$ agonists do not work significantly under the age of 2 years.
B   atopy is not necessarily a cardinal feature of asthma.
C   in the treatment of an acute attack, intravenous hydrocortisone works more rapidly than oral prednisolone.
D   daily peak flow monitoring is a vital part of management in most children with asthma.
E   approximately 1% of the adult population have asthma.

**D14   Regarding child protection procedures:**
A   children can only be taken into care because of positive acts of abuse, not because of acts of omission.
B   it is the responsibility of social services to decide whether a child should be taken into long-term care.
C   Care Orders cannot be applied for simply because of the possibility of 'future harm'
D   psychiatric treatment for the emotional sequelae of child sexual abuse has to be deferred until after criminal proceedings are complete, as such treatment can compromise the giving of evidence.

**E** parents can be excluded from a case conference if their presence is considered to be against the child's interests.

**D15** **Classical features of a child with Noonan syndrome include:**
**A** short stature.
**B** coarctation of the aorta.
**C** polydactyly.
**D** cryptorchidism.
**E** deafness.

**D16** **The following are true of Wolff–Parkinson–White syndrome (WPW):**
**A** there is a short P-R interval.
**B** the arrhythmia associated with this syndrome is irregular.
**C** the frequency of attacks characteristically reduces as the child grows older.
**D** digoxin is the drug of choice for prophylaxis.
**E** electrical cardioversion should precede drug treatment in an attack.

**D17** **In chronic granulomatous disease (CGD):**
**A** functions of B and T lymphocytes are markedly impaired.
**B** prophylactic antibiotics are indicated.
**C** fungal infections are common.
**D** serum IgG levels are markedly increased.
**E** the basic problem is a defect in the alternative complement pathway.

**D18** **Regarding hyaline membrane disease (HMD):**
**A** can occur in infants of diabetic mothers of 37–40 weeks' gestation.
**B** infants born to mothers who are heroin addicts are at increased risk of HMD.
**C** a light-for-dates infant of 33 weeks' gestation has a greater risk of developing HMD than a 33-week infant of appropriate weight.
**D** administration of artificial surfactant is curative.
**E** chest X-ray findings are markedly different between cases of HMD and Group B streptococcal pneumonia.

**D19** **Autism:**
**A** is a condition in which it is desirable to keep affected children in mainstream schools.
**B** can occur in children who have shown normal development for the first four years of life.
**C** characteristically affects linguistic communication while sparing non-verbal communication.
**D** characteristically occurs in children of above average IQ.
**E** is thought to be the result of extreme deprivation.

**D20** **Lowe syndrome (oculocerebrorenal syndrome):**

**A** may present with aminoaciduria.
**B** is inherited as an autosomal recessive.
**C** characteristically has stippling of patellae on X-ray.
**D** may present with cataracts.
**E** commonly progresses to renal failure in adolescence.

# PAPER D
## ANSWERS

**D1**    **A**    **False**    Although a brain tumour may present in an infant with a large and increasing head size, once the sutures have closed brain tumours usually present with classic symptoms and signs of raised intracranial pressure (headache, vomiting, VIth nerve palsies and papilloedema).

      **B**    **False**    Most brain tumours in childhood are infratentorial, the commonest being the medulloblastoma.

      **C**    **True**    Deteriorating school performance and/or personality change in the absence of other signs may be due to slow-growing tumours in the frontal lobes.

      **D**    **False**    While 25% of adult brain tumours are metastatic the figure is much lower in childhood (<5%).

      **E**    **False**    Even 'benign' (i.e. low grade) brain tumours are most often best treated as they will eventually cause problems (epilepsy, raised intracranial pressure).

**D2**    **A**    **True**

      **B**    **True**

      **C**    **True**    They all arise as a result of an expansion in a trinucleotide repeat sequence.

      **D**    **True**

      **E**    **False**    The figure is 100%.

**D3**    **A**    **False**    The primary renal lesion is Fanconi syndrome due to proximal tubular cell dysfunction. This leads to a failure to reabsorb potassium, bicarbonate and phosphate in the proximal tubule with their being wasted into the urine leading to low levels.

**B** **True** The gradual failure of proximal tubular function leads to delivery of more sodium distally than can be handled by the tubules and hence to polyuria. This usually leads to such severe polydipsia that children are not interested in eating, but drink almost non-stop.

**C** **True** This is multifactorial. The hypophosphataemia from hyperphosphaturia is an important cause as is the failure of 1 alpha hydroxylation of vitamin $D_3$ which occurs in the proximal tubule cell.

**D** **True** Cystine is taken up in the lysosomes of all metabolically active cells in the body where it forms crystals. Within the bone marrow these can be identified readily by polarized light. Though the bone marrow gives an instant result, an alternative diagnostic test is to measure the cystine concentration in white cells in peripheral blood. Cystine crystals become visible in the cornea using slit-lamp examination, and this is a useful test over the age of a year.

**E** **True** Cystine crystals accumulate in all metabolically active cells and hence the endocrine system is highly vulnerable.

**D4** **A** **True**

**B** **False** A cystic fibrosis sufferer *will* be at risk of night cramps in tropical Africa, but this will be due to *sodium* depletion due to excessive loss of sodium in sweat.

**C** **False**

**D** **False** While such a level is abnormal and suggestive of cystic fibrosis, sweat tests are notoriously variable and can be misleading. A definitive diagnosis should not be made on a single result of this level.

**E** **False**

**D5** **A** **False** The risk from various studies comes out at a fairly constant 40–45%.

**B** **True** This 40–45% risk certainly merits counselling against risky activities (cycling in traffic, swimming unsupervised, having deep baths, etc.). It is usual *not* to prescribe long-term anticonvulsants at this stage, but it would be perfectly reasonable to do so if there were a strong parental preference for treatment.

**C** **False** CT scanning is only warranted if there is clinical or EEG evidence of focality or abnormal physical findings.

**D** **False** 3 Hz spike and wave activity is characteristic of childhood absence epilepsy.

**E** **True** The combination of partial seizures involving the mouth with generalized tonic-clonic seizures suggests benign partial epilepsy of childhood ('Rolandic epilepsy'). This is one of the commonest childhood epilepsy syndromes and as its name implies has a high chance of spontaneous remission.

**D6** **A** **False** There is strong evidence from longitudinal studies that temperament at birth correlates well with later personality.

**B** **False** Parent–infant bonding is thought to occur maximally at this time. However, the infant is essentially too undifferentiated to reciprocate equally. *Attachment* behaviour (infant to parent) begins around 6 months of age (with the infant resisting separation), and develops with increasing intensity to a peak at 18–24 months.

**C** **True** Latency is a very useful concept in which the child 'coasts' or 'freewheels' without worrying too much about big issues like life and death. He or she just 'gets on with life'.

**D** **False** See (B). A one-week separation for a 2-year-old child can be a seriously traumatic event unless a loving substitute parent is provided. A 3-month baby is paradoxically more resilient, because less differentiated.

**E** **True** Erikson postulated 8 stages to cover the entire lifespan.

**D7** **A** **False** Sarcoidosis characteristically causes uveitis. Tuberculosis causes a phlyctenular conjunctivitis.

**B** **True** This is the commonest presentation of the condition, usually associated with hilar lymphadenopathy and lung parenchymal changes on chest X-ray.

**C** **True** This can be bilateral, especially in association with parotitis.

**D** **True** In association with uveitis the term uveo-parotid fever has been used.

**E** **True** This is usually mild.

**D8 A True** Maternal immunity is humoral, and immunity to pertussis is cellular. Infants can catch pertussis in the first week of life.

**B True** While lymphocytosis in the first week would support the diagnosis it is not definitive. Likewise positive bacteriological culture is only found in 40% of clinical cases. The diagnosis should be made on the *history* of the cough, in which there should be prolonged bouts of coughing (30–60 seconds), and the cough should have a staccato or machine gun-like character with few pauses for inspiration. A whoop is an optional extra and is often absent in the infant under a year of age (the time at which the disease carries a risk of mortality from apnoea).

**C False** See (B).

**D False** See (B)

**E False** The duration is usually around 3 months (in China it is called 'the 100 day cough'). Subsequent viral URTIs can appear to trigger a brief relapse.

**D9 A False** ADHD has long been recognized in Australian and American paediatrics but has only recently become a respectable diagnosis in the UK. Best estimates suggest a population incidence of between 1 and 5 *per cent* making it one of the 'top ten' conditions of childhood.

**B False** A significant number of cases carry their handicap into adult life. Having said that, children who have responded well to good early management (often with amphetamines) may be weaned off medication in adolescence because they have gained better coping strategies during the years of treatment.

**C True** Such children are at extra high risk of school failure especially if undiagnosed. The effects on peer relationships and self-esteem increase the risk of antisocial behaviour.

**D False** ADHD is thought to arise from genetic rather than environmental factors and as such is probably distributed evenly through all social classes. However, as with dyslexia, the chances of being diagnosed and treated are naturally higher for children in the higher social classes.

**E True** The other features are hyperactivity and short concentration span. Oppositional and defiant behaviour with or without an insatiable quality may also be seen.

**D10** **A** **False** Pulsus paradoxus is important clinical evidence that an attack is severe. It is due to an exaggeration (not in fact paradoxical) of the reduction in cardiac output during inspiration. This is normally due to reduced venous return to the left side of the heart. In severe asthma the normal increase in venous return to the right side of the heart is obstructed by the increased intrathoracic pressure, and this accentuates the fall in pulse volume during inspiration.

**B** **False** The fear of oxygen concentrations above 40% is mainly relevant to adult patients with chronic hypercapnia whose respiratory drive depends on hypoxia. This situation would be extremely rare in childhood asthma, and in general children should receive as high a concentration of $O_2$ as they require to maintain a satisfactory $Po_2$.

**C** **False** Although this form of treatment is surprisingly common it is essentially irrational. Hydrocortisone is not a bronchodilator but an anti-inflammatory drug, and the sooner the total dose is inside the body the better.

**D** **False** While this statement sounds plausible/praiseworthy, many children with this level of $Pco_2$ can pull through without and clinical judgement can be allowed some latitude in this decision.

**E** **False** Ventilating a severe asthmatic can be quite challenging and is completely different from the situation in, for example, hyaline membrane disease. Because the main problem is air trapping, slow rates with long expiratory times are required.

**D11** **A** **False** The figure is more than 2000 ml.

**B** **True**

**C** **False** Renal agenesis (as in Potter syndrome) is associated with *oligo*hydrammios, due to the absence of urinary output.

**D** **True** Due to decreased fetal ability to swallow amniotic fluid.

**E** **True**

**D12** **A** **True** The two main haemoglobinopathies are the thalassaemias and sickle cell disease.

**B** **False** Congenital spherocytosis is due to an inherited abnormality of the red cell membrane.

C   **False**   Pyruvate kinase deficiency is a rare example of a red cell enzyme defect. It is inherited as an autosomal recessive and causes a chronic haemolytic anaemia.

D   **False**

E   **True**   See (A).

**D13**   A   **False**   While this is mildly controversial, current majority opinion would be that $\beta_2$ agonists *do* work significantly in this age group, albeit sometimes to a lesser extent than in older children.

B   **True**   Again mildly debatable, but current usage of the word asthma regards atopic asthma as just one variety of asthma. Bronchial hyperreactivity to a variety of stimuli (not only allergens) is regarded as the cardinal feature of asthma.

C   **False**   In the absence of vomiting, both therapies work at roughly the same rate, producing clinical improvement in 1–3 hours (admittedly the study was done in adults).

D   **False**   This statement is too extreme and ignores the facts that (i) it is inappropriate for pre-school children and (ii) it is a waste of time for most mild or episodic asthmatics.

E   **False**   The figure is nearer to 5%.

**D14**   A   **False**   Under the Children Act 1989, Care Orders can be granted because of acts of commission *or* omission that cause or are likely to cause 'significant harm'. Prior to this, the key phrase was that 'the child's proper development was being avoidably impaired'.

B   **False**   The final responsibility lies with the courts, to which the social services must apply.

C   **False**   Children do not have to be harmed before they can be protected. Indeed, children can be taken into care at birth.

D   **False**   Despite the risk of compromising evidence, the Official Solicitor has deemed that it is bad practice to withhold treatment.

E   **True**   However, in the author's experience this clause is rarely invoked, and parents are only excluded if they have a past history of violence to a professional!

**D15**  A  **True**
    B  **False**    Pulmonary stenosis is the classic heart defect. ASD is also common.

    C  **False**
    D  **True**
    E  **True**

**D16**  A  **True**    This is due to the broadening of the QRS complex due to the delta wave at the beginning, which is the cardinal feature of this condition.

    B  **False**    The arrhythmia associated with WPW syndrome is paroxysmal supraventricular tachycardia (SVT), which is a *regular* arrhythmia, with a rate of c.300/min.

    C  **True**
    D  **False**    While digoxin is still used in the prophylaxis of SVT, it is relatively contraindicated if there is underlying WPW syndrome.

    E  **False**    In SVT, vagal stimulation should be tried first, *then* drug treatment (IV adenosine), *then* electrical cardioversion.

**D17**  A  **False**    In this rare condition, the basic defect is in the ability of polymorphonuclear neutrophils to kill phagocytosed bacteria and fungi, which therefore cause granulomata in lymph nodes. Humoral immunity and lymphocytic function is unaffected. Most cases occur in boys, suggesting an X-linked mode of inheritance. The diagnostic test is the NBT (nitroblue tetrazolium) test.

    B  **True**    There is increasing evidence that interferon is also beneficial.

    C  **True**
    D  **True**    Presumably in response to the high load of bacterial antigen in the body.

    E  **False**    See (A).

**D18**  A  **True**    This is thought to be due to delayed synthesis of surfactant.

    B  **False**    While the infants may be more 'at risk' in other ways, the risk of HMD is actually reduced in infants of heroin addicts, probably because heroin increases lung maturation.

| | | | |
|---|---|---|---|
| | C | False | The stress of being light for dates seems to enhance lung maturation and protect from HMD. |
| | D | False | Artificial surfactant is best regarded as effective supportive treatment which reduces the severity of HMD without abolishing it completely. |
| | E | False | While most other bacteria causing congenital pneumonia characteristically cause patchy or streaky opacities, Group B streptococcal infection gives a classic groundglass appearance indistinguishable from HMD. |
| D19 | A | False | Autism is a rare (1:10 000) severely handicapping condition in which a severe language disorder coexists with profound abnormalities in relating to other people. It is probably genetic in origin and is almost certainly not due to an abnormal early environment. About two thirds of autistic children will have severe learning disability, and nearly all will need early placement in a special school. |
| | B | False | First symptoms are virtually always apparent within the first three years of life. |
| | C | False | All forms of social relationships and communication are affected. |
| | D | False | See (A). |
| | E | False | See (A). |
| D20 | A | True | This is a rare X-linked recessive condition presenting with cataracts and/or glaucoma in infancy and subsequent severe mental retardation. |
| | B | False | See (A). |
| | C | False | This is a feature of Zellweger syndrome (cerebrohepatorenal syndrome). |
| | D | True | See (A). |
| | E | False | The renal anomaly only affects tubular function, with tubular proteinuria and aminoaciduria without progression to renal failure. |

# PAPER E
## QUESTIONS

**E1** The following are recognized features of the mucocutaneous lymph node syndrome (Kawasaki disease):
A aneurysms of the coronary arteries.
B cervical lymphadenopathy.
C arthritis.
D treatment with immunoglobulin within the first 10 days of onset is desirable.
E aseptic meningitis.

**E2** The following statements are correct regarding asthma in childhood:
A approximately 5% of children develop asthma at some stage in their childhood.
B most severely asthmatic children begin to wheeze during the first year of life.
C children who wheeze only in response to viral infections do not respond to bronchodilators.
D roughly 1% of children continue to suffer from asthma in adult life.
E the number of childhood deaths per year from asthma has fallen over the last 10 years.

**E3** Intussusception in childhood:
A consists most commonly of ileocaecal and ileocolic forms.
B occurs most commonly between the ages of 2 and 5 years.
C characteristically gives rise to a mass in the right iliac fossa.
D should always be treated surgically.
E abdominal X-ray characteristically shows gas in the wall of the affected bowel.

**E4** In the examination of the cranial nerves:
A an ipsilateral cranial nerve lesion with a contralateral hemiplegia suggests a lesion in the brain stem.
B unilateral upper motor neuron lesions of the XIIth cranial nerve are not clinically detectable.
C a bitemporal hemianopia suggests a lesion in the optic radiation.
D a lesion of the IVth cranial nerve causes a lateral rectus palsy.
E loss of taste to the anterior two thirds of the tongue can occur in lesions of the VIIth cranial nerve.

**E5**   **Features of the histiocytosis X group of conditions include:**
A   early age of onset carries a better prognosis.
B   osteolytic skull lesions on X-ray.
C   polyuria and polydipsia.
D   chronic maculopapular skin eruption.
E   hepatosplenomegaly.

**E6**   **A head circumference above the 97th centile:**
A   may be normal in a child whose height and weight are on the 50th centile.
B   is characteristic of the congenital rubella syndrome.
C   if found in conjunction with fundal haemorrhages in a 6-month-old infant, is likely to be secondary to *Haemophilus* meningitis.
D   may be associated with the Arnold–Chiari malformation.
E   may be a feature of cerebral gigantism.

**E7**   **Recognized complications of varicella include:**
A   pneumonia.
B   thrombocytopenia.
C   erythema marginatum.
D   parotitis.
E   otitis media.

**E8**   **The following are contraindications to specific immunizations:**
A   hypersensitivity to horse serum — tetanus toxoid.
B   a history of febrile convulsions — measles vaccination.
C   cystic fibrosis — pertussis vaccination.
D   concurrent antibiotic therapy — triple vaccination.
E   eczema — pertussis vaccination.

**E9**   **In kwashiorkor:**
A   there is a significant risk of hypothermia.
B   the disease occurs only in children below the 50th centile for weight.
C   the incidence is highest in the first year of life.
D   the disease may be precipitated by measles.
E   cardiac failure may occur during the initial stages of treatment.

**E10**   **A child is found to have lost some previously documented skills:**
A   the child has a progressive neurological condition.
B   childhood progressive encephalopathies are genetic.
C   if the aetiology cannot be identified, autosomal recessive inheritance should be assumed in genetic counselling.
D   progressive encephalopathies may be missed in very young children.
E   no progressive brain pathology may be identifiable.

**E11** The following malformations can occur in children born to mothers who have insulin-dependent diabetes mellitus:
A cleft lip/palate.
B caudal regression syndrome.
C femoral hypoplasia.
D holoprosencephaly.
E polydactyly.

**E12** The following physical signs may be present in pericardial effusion:
A pulsatile liver.
B pulsus paradoxus.
C giant 'a' waves in the neck veins.
D a left parasternal heave.
E a loud first sound at the apex.

**E13** In a child with suspected liver disease, the following signs suggest impaired hepatocellular function:
A palmar erythema.
B splenomegaly.
C spider naevi.
D muscle wasting.
E visual hallucinations.

**E14** The following symptoms in an infant in the first month of life should alert one to the possibility of hypothyroidism:
A prolonged jaundice.
B vomiting.
C diarrhoea.
D hoarse cry.
E voracious appetite.

**E15** Regarding sickle cell anaemia:
A a positive sickling test is diagnostic of sickle cell disease.
B roughly 5% of Africans are carriers of the sickle cell trait.
C the heterozygous condition is usually asymptomatic.
D treatment with desferrioxamine has significantly improved the life expectancy in sickle cell disease.
E there is an increased predisposition to salmonella osteomyelitis.

**E16** In acute post-streptococcal glomerulonephritis:
A long-term prophylaxis with penicillin is indicated to prevent recurrence.
B there is usually a good response to a short course of high-dose prednisolone.
C most cases recover completely.
D there may be polyuria during the recovery phase.
E albumin infusion is seldom indicated for peripheral oedema.

**E17** **The following statements concerning childhood accidents are correct:**

    **A** they are commoner in boys than in girls.

    **B** they come second to neoplasia as a cause of death in the 1–4-year age group.

    **C** use of child-resistant containers can reduce the incidence of accidental ingestion of medicaments by toddlers.

    **D** gastric lavage is essential in all cases of suspected drug ingestion.

    **E** drug treatment for nocturnal enuresis carries some risk.

**E18** **The following statements about Down syndrome are true:**

    **A** there is a recognized association with duodenal atresia.

    **B** most cases are due to chromosomal translocation.

    **C** patients with near-normal IQs are usually cases of mosaicism.

    **D** the incidence is related to maternal age in cases due to translocation.

    **E** the incidence is related to paternal age in cases due to non-disjunction.

**E19** **The following are characteristic features of the mucosal neuronal syndrome:**

    **A** abnormal facies.

    **B** constipation.

    **C** familial tendency.

    **D** association with medullary carcinoma of the thyroid.

    **E** raised calcitonin levels.

**E20** **In the assessment and management of epilepsy in childhood:**

    **A** a normal EEG will exclude the diagnosis in a clinically doubtful case.

    **B** intramuscular diazepam is more effective than rectal diazepam in the treatment of status epilepticus.

    **C** sodium valproate has been associated with liver damage.

    **D** phenytoin can cause rickets.

    **E** petit mal is characterized by retrograde amnesia.

# PAPER E
## ANSWERS

**E1**  **A**  **True**  Kawasaki disease is an unusual condition which was initially reported widely in Japanese children but is increasingly being recognized in Europe and America. The aetiology is uncertain but it may be rickettsial infection. In a typical case there is prolonged fever and malaise with a generalized marked erythematous rash especially affecting the palms and soles. There is stomatitis, episcleritis and arthritis, and cases are commonly misdiagnosed as either the Stevens–Johnson syndrome or scarlet fever. Cervical lymphadenopathy is another basic feature of the disease and the ESR is usually very high. A virtually diagnostic feature of the condition is peeling of the skin of the hands during the convalescent period, which starts at the edges of the finger nails. A small proportion of cases (1–3%) suffer sudden death due to cardiac arrest during convalescence, and this has been found to be due to aneurysms and thromboses of the coronary arteries.

    **B**  **True**  See (A).

    **C**  **True**  See (A).

    **D**  **True**  This treatment significantly reduces the incidence of coronary aneurysms. Unfortunately, the diagnosis is often not made until 2–3 weeks into the illness. Low-dose aspirin for 6–12 months is recommended for cases with coronary aneurysms.

    **E**  **True**  Aseptic meningitis is a recognized feature of Kawasaki disease.

**E2**  **A**  **False**  The epidemiology of asthma has been a somewhat confused area in the past due to the use of differing terminology and definitions. It is now generally agreed that there is no justification for continuing to regard 'wheezy bronchitis' as a different disease entity, but to regard children previously given this label as part of the spectrum of asthma. Using this view, it is found that 15–20% of children suffer from significant asthma during their childhood, and there is naturally a wide range of severity contained within these figures. Most children grow out of their asthma during childhood, but up to 5% (of all children) may go on wheezing significantly as they enter adult life.

    **B**  **True**  The converse, however, does not necessarily hold; i.e. many children who wheeze in their first year of life do not necessarily develop severe asthma.

    **C**  **False**  There is no clinically significant evidence for this view, although it might be true of a small number of individual children in the younger age groups.

    **D**  **False**  The figure is nearer 5%, see (A).

    **E**  **False**  While numbers are hard to come by, it seems that, surprisingly, the great improvements in available treatment over the past 10 years have not been applied in such a way as to significantly affect mortality from asthma, which has probably continued to the order of 50–100 children per year over this period.

**E3**  **A**  **True**  The ileum is the portion of bowel most commonly involved at the apex of an intussusception. The precipitating cause may be lymphoid hyperplasia in a Peyer's patch.

    **B**  **False**  Over 75% of cases present under the age of 2 years.

    **C**  **False**  The right iliac fossa usually feels 'empty' and the mass if present is most commonly felt in the right hypochondrium.

    **D**  **False**  While some cases will require surgery, in quite a significant number surgery can be avoided by successful hydrostatic reduction by a barium enema.

    **E**  **False**  Intramural bowel gas is a characteristic finding in advanced cases of necrotizing enterocolitis (NEC), a disease of neonates carrying a high mortality and morbidity. It is not a feature of the X-ray in intussusception; instead the characteristic finding is of *absence* of gas in the right iliac fossa.

**E4**   **A**   **True**   A unilateral brain stem lesion may involve a cranial nerve nucleus and the corticospinal tract. The latter will supply the opposite side of the body after crossing at the decussation of the pyramids. The cranial nerve lesion will be ipsilateral (i.e. on the same side as the lesion) because the cortical fibres supplying it have already crossed, and the hemiplegia will be contralateral. A 'crossed paralysis' of this type is diagnostic of a brain stem lesion.

**B**   **True**   Most cranial nerves, including the XIIth, have bilateral cortical innervation and therefore unilateral cortical lesions do not produce clinical signs. Exceptions to this rule are the XIth cranial nerve, and that portion of the VIIth which supplies the lower portion of the face. Bilateral cortical lesions are necessary to produce (bilateral) upper motor neuron lesions of the cranial nerves and this clinical syndrome is known as pseudobulbar palsy.

**C**   **False**   Bitemporal hemianopia is a sign of involvement of the optic chiasm, e.g. by a pituitary tumour such as a craniopharyngioma. Lesions of the optic radiation give an homonymous hemianopia, often quadrantic.

**D**   **False**   The lateral rectus is supplied by the VIth cranial nerve, the IVth supplying the superior oblique. The VIth cranial nerve is liable to be affected by raised intracranial pressure which may itself be due to a lesion elsewhere. In this event the VIth nerve palsy is a 'false localizing sign'.

**E**   **True**   Taste sensation to the anterior two thirds of the tongue is carried via the chorda tympani, which is part of the intrapetrous portion of the VIIth cranial nerve. The chorda tympani leaves the facial nerve just before the latter exits through the stylomastoid foramen. Lesions of the facial nerve proximal to this point can therefore cause loss of taste sensation to the anterior two thirds of the tongue.

**E5**   **A**   **False**   Early age of onset is usual in the most severe form of this condition (Letterer–Siwe disease). The mildest form of the condition, eosinophilic granuloma, characteristically occurs in older children.

**B**   **True**   Osteolytic lesions of bone, especially the skull, are characteristic in histiocytosis X.

**C** **True** Diabetes insipidus is a characteristic feature of the variety of histiocytosis X known as Hand–Schüller–Christian disease. Other features include proptosis, skin rashes and honeycomb lung.

**D** **True** A chronic seborrhoeic rash is a common feature of Letterer–Siwe disease.

**E** **True** Hepatosplenomegaly with lymphadenopathy, failure to thrive and pyrexia are typical features of Letterer–Siwe disease.

**E6** **A** **True** The usual cause of this situation is a familial pattern of large heads.

**B** **False** Congenital rubella causes microcephaly.

**C** **False** The most likely cause of this combination of signs would be non-accidental injury (shaking) leading to subdural haematoma and fundal haemorrhages.

**D** **True** The Arnold–Chiari malformation consists of hypoplasia of the cerebellum with herniation of the cerebellar tonsils through the foramen magnum. It is a characteristic finding in the hydrocephalus found with neural tube defects. Whether it is a cause or a result of hydrocephalus is still unclear, with majority opinion appearing to favour the latter.

**E** **True** In cerebral gigantism (Soto syndrome) there is a combination of large head, somatic gigantism, abnormal facies and mental retardation.

**E7** **A** **True** Varicella is usually a mild disease in childhood, and like most exanthems can be more severe in the non-immune adult. An interstitial pneumonia is a recognized complication and can result in subsequent diffuse calcification on chest X-ray. This complication is more likely to occur in adults.

**B** **False** Thrombocytopenia is a complication of rubella.

**C** **False** Erythema marginatum is characteristic of acute rheumatic fever.

**D** **False** Parotitis is the hallmark of mumps.

**E** **False** Otitis media is a common complication of measles.

**E8**  **A**  **False**  Tetanus antitoxin (ATS) of equine origin was once used in the management of a case of tetanus if human immune globulin was unavailable. However, this is nothing to do with tetanus toxoid which has no constituents of equine origin. Accordingly hypersensitivity to horse serum does not contraindicate a course of tetanus toxoid.

**B**  **False**  Measles vaccine being a live vaccine may cause a mild measles-like illness after 7–10 days, and this might possibly cause a further febrile convulsion. However, the risks of a convulsion would be considerably higher with proper measles, and vaccine should still be offered with suitable advice on temperature control.

**C**  **False**  Cystic fibrosis constitutes a strong indication for pertussis vaccination as a combination of the two diseases could be most unpleasant for the child.

**D**  **False**  While it is currently orthodox to withhold triple vaccine during 'the acute phase of a febrile illness', the subsequent completion of a course of antibiotics is no reason for further postponement.

**E**  **False**  There is a widespread myth that eczema is a strong contraindication to immunization against pertussis. This is not the case, and the only vaccination for which eczema constitutes a contraindication is smallpox, which is not on routine offer nowadays anyway.

**E9**  **A**  **True**  This complication is thought to be due to failure of enzymes limiting the metabolic response to cold.

**B**  **False**  Kwashiorkor is a condition produced by a severe dietary deficiency of protein and in developing countries typically follows a significant environmental change such as the arrival of a further baby or a change of caretaker. Even a previously well-nourished infant on the 97th centile for weight can be precipitated into kwashiorkor by such events if they result in, for example, sudden cessation of breast feeding with 'promotion' to a diet consisting almost entirely of carbohydrate. The environmental change is frequently accompanied by deterioration in the emotional warmth the child experiences, and this may secondarily lead to anorexia.

**C   False**   The incidence is commonest in the second and third years of life because this is the stage at which the child is most often displaced by a new sibling or sent to a new caretaker.

**D   True**   Measles can lead to a severe reduction in dietary intake associated with gastrointestinal upset. If cultural beliefs preclude adequate feeding during the illness this combination can be a precipitant of kwashiorkor.

**E   True**   Anaemia may be a complicating factor in any type of malnutrition, and this may contribute to the causation of cardiac failure. The main mechanisms thought to be responsible are:

(i)   cardiac muscle dysfunction, and

(ii)   hypervolaemia due to return of oedema fluid to the vascular compartment as the serum albumin rises.

**E10   A   False**   Developmental regression is a very important neurological syndrome, and should always alert one to the possibility of a progressive encephalopathy (often with a metabolic basis). However, subclinical epilepsy and drugs are two important treatable causes that need to be considered.

**B   False**   Most childhood encephalopathies are genetic. Exceptions include subacute viral encephalopathies (SSPE, HIV) and progressive anatomical problems (hydrocephalus, space-occupying lesion).

**C   False**   Most progressive encephalopathies are autosomal recessive, but a few are X-linked.

**D   True**   This is because they have not had time to acquire skills sufficient to demonstrate regression.

**E   True**   Some children with autism may show regression without demonstrable evidence of brain pathology.

**E11   A   False**

**B   True**

**C   True**

**D   True**

**E   True**

**E12** **A** **False**  Whilst the liver is commonly enlarged due to venous congestion in pericardial effusion, it will not be pulsatile. A pulsatile liver occurs in tricuspid incompetence and in hepatic arteriovenous malformation.

**B** **True**  Pulsus paradoxus is a sign of cardiac tamponade and can occur in both pericardial effusion and constrictive pericarditis. It also occurs in conditions associated with increased intrathoracic pressure such as severe asthma. Pulsus paradoxus consists of a diminution in the pulse volume during inspiration, and is not in fact paradoxical but an exaggeration of normal changes.

**C** **False**  The jugular venous pressure may be raised in pericardial effusion but the distended veins will show normal pulsation. Giant 'a' waves are a sign of right atrial hypertrophy.

**D** **False**  The cardiac impulse from both ventricles is 'damped down' in pericardial effusion. A left parasternal heave is evidence of right ventricular hypertrophy, which is not present in uncomplicated pericardial effusion.

**E** **False**  Both heart sounds are muffled in pericardial effusion. A loud first sound is characteristic in mitral stenosis, being due to the mitral valve closing against increased left atrial pressure.

**E13** **A** **True**  Palmar erythema is thought to be due to impaired hepatic breakdown of endogenous oestrogens, and is a recognized sign of impaired hepatocellular function.

**B** **False**  Splenomegaly secondary to liver disease is a sign of portal hypertension, not impaired hepatocellular function.

**C** **True**  Spider naevi, like palmar erythema, are signs of increased circulating oestrogens.

**D** **True**  In advanced cases of hepatocellular failure, impaired hepatic synthesis of protein leads to muscle wasting, usually together with significant hypoalbuminaemia and oedema.

**E** **True**  Visual hallucinations are characteristic of a toxic confusional state (organic psychosis) and advanced hepatocellular failure can cause the latter (hepatic encephalopathy). Auditory hallucinations are extremely rare in childhood and are a sign of true psychosis.

**E14**  **A  True**    Prolonged jaundice may be due to breast milk jaundice or neonatal hepatitis/biliary atresia, among other causes. However, it should always lead to the early investigation of thyroid function, as it is a common feature of hypothyroidism, and early diagnosis and treatment are so important.

  **B  False**    Vomiting is not a recognized feature of congenital hypothyroidism. Infants may be poor feeders and fail to thrive.

  **C  False**    Hypothyroidism at any age causes constipation, not diarrhoea.

  **D  True**    There are many similarities between the clinical features of congenital and adult hypothyroidism. One of these is the abnormally hoarse voice which is a feature of both conditions.

  **E  False**    As already stated, hypothyroid infants tend to be poor feeders and fail to thrive.

**E15**  **A  False**    The sickling test (which consists of adding sodium metabisulphite to blood) is positive in both sickle cell disease and sickle cell trait. A more discriminating test is simply to look at the blood film, which is normal in sickle cell trait but may show spontaneous sickling in the homozygote. The definitive investigation is haemoglobin electrophoresis.

  **B  False**    The figure is nearer to 15%.

  **C  True**    However, problems may arise with low oxygen tension due, for example, to high altitude or general anaesthesia.

  **D  False**    There is no specific treatment for sickle cell disease, and management is mainly supportive. (A few severe cases have benefited from bone marrow transplantation.) Folate supplements may be indicated in the prevention or treatment of aplastic crises. Desferrioxamine is a chelating agent for the treatment of iron overload, and is mainly used for this purpose in cases of beta thalassaemia, who require far more frequent transfusions than patients with sickle cell disease.

  **E  True**    Other predispositions include pneumococcal septicaemia and aseptic necrosis of the femoral head.

**E16**  **A**  **False**  Long-term penicillin prophylaxis is recommended in cases of rheumatic fever, which can relapse following infection with *any* β-haemolytic streptococcus. However, glomerulonephritis is only associated with infection by a few specific types of streptococcus (especially Type 12) and these are so rare as to render prophylaxis unnecessary. Of course, the precipitating streptococcal infection should be eradicated by a 10-day course of penicillin.

 **B**  **False**  Steroid therapy has no effect on the disease process in post-streptococcal glomerulonephritis, and management consists of eradication of the streptococcus together with medical management of any degree of renal failure that may occur.

 **C**  **True**  Most cases (over 95%) of post-streptococcal glomerulonephritis recover completely. A very small number may succumb to acute renal failure and its complications, and the remainder may present later with chronic renal failure or the nephrotic syndrome.

 **D**  **True**  After a period of anuria or oliguria, glomerular filtration often increases rapidly while tubular function is slower to recover. This may result in a marked diuretic phase during recovery from glomerulonephritis, during which large quantities of fluid and electrolytes are lost which need to be replaced.

 **E**  **True**  Any peripheral oedema occurring in acute glomerulonephritis is due to water overload as a result of renal failure. It is not due to hypoproteinaemia which, of course, is a cardinal feature of the nephrotic syndrome. Accordingly, albumin infusions are not indicated in acute glomerulonephritis, and they could in fact be harmful by exacerbating hypervolaemia. However, in a minority of cases of post-streptococcal glomerulonephritis, there is an additional nephrotic element and in these cases albumin might be indicated.

**E17**  **A**  **True**  Most types of accident are commoner in boys than girls, especially road traffic accidents. It would seem that at present boys are more likely to have accidents than girls because they are more prone to exploratory, hyperactive or impulsive behaviour.

**B  False**   Accidents are by far the commonest cause of death in children after the first year of life, and this is true from the ages of 1 to 14. Road accidents are the commonest accidental cause of death followed by drowning and burns. Neoplasia causes less than half the number of fatalities that are caused by accidents.

**C  True**   Initial evidence of the beneficial effect of child-resistant containers came from studies in service encampments in the USA. Since the introduction of child-resistant containers in the UK there has been a fall in the incidence of childhood poisoning due to drugs.

**D  False**   Gastric lavage is rarely indicated in children, its use being limited to the unconscious patient who has a cuffed endotracheal tube in place. In other situations where it is desirable to empty the stomach of an ingested substance, induced emesis is far preferable on the grounds of efficacy and of humanity. The drug of choice is probably syrup of ipecacuanha. The continuing popularity of gastric lavage in adult medical practice seems to be based on punitive intent rather than any medical reason.

**E  True**   The commonest drugs used in the treatment of enuresis are imipramine and amitriptyline. These are extremely dangerous drugs which can cause death from cardiac arrhythmias if taken in overdose. Ingestion by young children in dangerous quantities is more likely if the drug is prescribed in syrup form.

**E18  A  True**

**B  False**   Over 90% of cases of Down syndrome are due to non-disjunction, about 6% are due to translocations and 2% to mosaicism.

**C  True**

**D  False**   Translocation cases are not associated with increased maternal age.

**E  False**   Non-disjunction is associated with increased *maternal* age, with an increasingly steep rise in incidence with ages of over 35 years.

**E19** **A** **True** This rare condition usually presents with a combination of failure to thrive, diarrhoea and an abnormal appearance, together with hypotonia and possible developmental delay. The abnormal facies includes thick eyelids, patulous lips and prognathism. There may be neuromas on the tongue, buccal mucosa, lips and conjunctivae, together with peripheral neurofibromata and café-au-lait spots. There is often associated phaeochromocytomas, hyperparathyroidism and medullary carcinoma of the thyroid. All these tumours are derived from neural crest tissue, and the whole syndrome is inherited, usually as a dominant, so relatives should be screened (by measuring serum calcitonin). The most serious part of the syndrome is the medullary carcinoma of the thyroid which, if present, will be an indication for thyroidectomy.

**B** **False** The condition characteristically causes diarrhoea, because of raised levels of prostaglandins and serotonin secreted by the tumour. The serum calcium is usually low owing to raised calcitonin levels. (It is theoretically possible for coexisting hyperparathyroidism to cause an elevation of the serum calcium which could lead to constipation but this would hardly be characteristic of the condition.)

**C** **True** See (A).

**D** **True**

**E** **True** The calcitonin level may be raised even if the medullary carcinoma of the thyroid is occult, and this test is used to screen relatives.

**E20** **A** **False** The EEG may be normal in definite clinical cases of grand mal epilepsy. Conversely, the EEG may be abnormal in children who have never had any seizures. EEG reports should always be interpreted with care and should not be allowed to override the clinical diagnosis.

**B    False**    Intramuscular diazepam is absorbed so unsatisfactorily that it is virtually contraindicated in the management of status epilepticus. Cautious intravenous diazepam is the ideal, but diazepam is well absorbed rectally and has been shown to produce therapeutic blood levels in 10–15 minutes. It is therefore reasonable for parents to be encouraged to use rectal diazepam in emergencies at home.

**C    True**    Sodium valproate has been associated with fatalities from liver failure. While the complication appears to be very rare, the manufacturers recommend that liver function tests be performed before and during the first 6 months of treatment. The commonest side effect of the drug is obesity; other rare complications include thrombocytopenia and pancreatitis.

**D    True**    Both phenytoin and phenobarbitone can cause rickets during prolonged use. The mechanism is thought to be by interference with the metabolism of vitamin D in the liver.

**E    False**    In petit mal epilepsy, there is characteristically amnesia for events occuring *during* the attack, but no amnesia for events immediately prior to the attack.

# PAPER F
## QUESTIONS

**F1** **A 1-year-old child is brought to casualty with a 2-day history of apparent pain in the left leg. Examination reveals a miserable child with bony tenderness over the upper end of the left tibia:**
- **A.** a normal X-ray will exclude osteitis.
- **B** if there has been delay in seeking treatment, this suggests the possibility of non-accidental injury.
- **C** if a diagnosis of osteitis is made, antibiotic treatment should be postponed until the result of blood culture is obtained.
- **D** a combination of penicillin and cloxacillin is the initial drug regimen of choice for osteitis while awaiting sensitivities.
- **E** bone marrow biopsy may be indicated despite a normal peripheral blood film.

**F2** **In the management of a child with meningococcal septicaemia:**
- **A** if the patient is in shock, 4% dextrose in 0.18% saline is the replacement fluid of choice.
- **B** penicillin therapy must be withheld until blood culture, CSF and throat swabs have been taken.
- **C** calculation of the infant's vascular compartment is based on the formula: 85 ml/kg.
- **D** the prognosis is better in children who present with meningitis.
- **E** the diagnosis of 'shock' depends on the demonstration of a low blood pressure.

**F3** **The following conditions predispose to cerebral abscess formation:**
- **A** skull fracture involving the frontal sinus.
- **B** suppurative lung disease.
- **C** viral meningitis.
- **D** congenital heart disease with a left-to-right shunt.
- **E** chronic middle-ear sepsis.

**F4** **The following are characteristic features of migraine:**
- **A** vasodilatation of cerebral vessels precedes vasoconstriction.
- **B** homonymous hemianopia may occur during prodromal phase.

C   there may be a past history of recurrent abdominal pain.
D   ergotamine preparations are especially useful in hemiplegic migraine.
E   in post-pubertal girls, attacks are especially common in mid-cycle.

**F5**   **With regard to respiratory distress syndrome (RDS) of the newborn:**
A   meconium aspiration pneumonia is especially likely to be the cause if the infant is preterm.
B   hyaline membrane disease (HMD) is unlikely to be the cause if prepartum lecithin: sphingomyelin (L:S) ratio in amniotic fluid is greater than 2:1.
C   patchy opacities on chest X-ray are evidence in favour of a diagnosis of hyaline membrane disease.
D   in the artificial ventilation of infants with hyaline membrane disease, inflation pressures must never exceed 30 cm of water.
E   continuous positive airway pressure (CPAP) is an effective treatment for pneumothorax.

**F6**   **The following are true of convulsions in the neonatal period:**
A   sodium valproate is the drug of choice.
B   convulsions may respond to injection of pyridoxine.
C   convulsions may present as apnoeic attacks.
D   the prognosis for normal development is poor in the majority of cases.
E   a history of maternal narcotic addiction may be relevant.

**F7**   **In examination of the cardiovascular system in childhood:**
A   a venous hum is best heard with the child lying flat.
B   ventricular septal defects may not be clinically detectable in the first few days of life.
C   intercostal recession is useful evidence for a left-to-right shunt.
D   normal femoral pulses at birth exclude coarctation of the aorta.
E   peripheral oedema is a valuable sign of heart failure in infancy.

**F8**   **In an acute attack of asthma not responding completely to a nebulized bronchodilator, accepted treatment includes:**
A   beclomethasone by inhalation.
B   a short course of oral prednisolone.
C   oral ketotifen.
D   oral propranolol.
E   intravenous aminophylline.

**F9** The following are recognized associations of Crohn's disease in childhood:
A arthritis.
B increased incidence of neoplasia of large bowel.
C finger clubbing.
D erythema nodosum.
E aphthous stomatitis.

**F10** The following investigations may be appropriate in a case of childhood cirrhosis:
A slit-lamp examination of the eyes.
B glycosylated haemoglobin.
C serum $\alpha_1$-antitrypsin level.
D urine for reducing substances.
E sweat test.

**F11** Recognized causes of a height below the 3rd centile in a 10-year-old child include:
A congenital adrenal hyperplasia.
B Crohn's disease.
C XXY karyotype.
D emotional deprivation.
E XO karyotype.

**F12** The following statements are true concerning the complications of treatment for acute lymphoblastic leukaemia in childhood.
A pneumonia due to *Pneumocystis carinii* is best treated with erythromycin.
B measles vaccine is contraindicated in children on maintenance therapy.
C growth hormone deficiency may occur as a result of cranial irradiation.
D female survivors are almost universally sterile.
E allopurinol should be given for the first year of maintenance treatment to reduce the risk of hyperuricaemia.

**F13** Concerning hereditary spherocytosis:
A presence of spherocytes in the neonatal period is diagnostic of this condition.
B inheritance is as an autosomal dominant.
C the direct Coombs' test is positive in more than 50% of cases.
D the condition may present as jaundice in the neonatal period.
E splenectomy reverses the tendency to form spherocytes.

**F14** In a child with possible urinary problems:
A absence of a good stream in a male infant suggests posterior urethral valves.

**B**   circumcision should be offered to boys whose prepuces do not retract by the second birthday.
**C**   nocturnal enuresis should be regarded as normal up to the age of 10 years.
**D**   double micturition raises the possibility of ureteric reflux.
**E**   a positive urine culture of 40 000 organisms/ml should be regarded as significant.

**F15   Human breast milk:**
**A**   is rich in secretory IgA.
**B**   is contraindicated in galactosaemia.
**C**   is contraindicated in hereditary fructose intolerance.
**D**   is produced in response to prolactin.
**E**   is low in phosphorus compared with cow's milk.

**F16   The following are characteristic features of a 4-year-old with deprivational dwarfism (psychosocial dwarfism, maternal deprivation syndrome, non-organic failure to thrive):**
**A**   infantile body proportions.
**B**   pot belly.
**C**   normal speech development.
**D**   marked separation anxiety on being left in hospital by parents.
**E**   affection-seeking behaviour.

**F17   The following observations would give serious grounds for concern in a 1-year-old baby:**
**A**   failure to pass a cube from hand to hand.
**B**   inability to stand without support.
**C**   inability to sit for 3 seconds.
**D**   no meaningful words other than 'mama' and 'dada'.
**E**   adapts easily to admission to hospital without mother.

**F18   The following signs are characteristic of ovarian dysgenesis (Turner syndrome):**
**A**   chromatin negative buccal smear.
**B**   clitoral hypertrophy.
**C**   oedema in the neonatal period.
**D**   syndactyly.
**E**   associated congenital heart disease.

**F19   The following conditions typically cause cerebellar ataxia in childhood:**
**A**   medulloblastoma.
**B**   meningioma of the falx cerebri.
**C**   polio.
**D**   varicella encephalitis.
**E**   dystonia musculorum deformans.

**F20** **The following are possible features of an intrinsic lesion of the spinal cord in the cervical region:**

**A** dissociated anaesthesia over the arms and shoulders.
**B** Horner syndrome.
**C** wasting of leg muscles.
**D** nystagmus.
**E** numbness over the lower face.

# PAPER F
## ANSWERS

**F1**

**A False** X-rays are usually normal in the early stages of osteitis, the characteristic changes of rarefaction and subperiosteal new bone formation not usually appearing for 10–14 days. Diagnosis and a decision to commence treatment should depend largely on clinical evidence, although a polymorphonuclear leukocytosis is useful additional evidence. A radio-isotope bone scan may show abnormality much earlier than an X-ray.

**B True** Delay in seeking appropriate medical treatment should always lead to a consideration of non-accidental injury as a diagnosis, especially in a young child whose symptoms could be due to trauma. However such delay is not certain evidence of non-accidental injury as there are other innocent reasons for delay in seeking medical help, e.g. fear of doctors and hospitals, wishful thinking that one's child is not really ill, etc. Conversely, some parents who have injured their children seek medical help without delay.

**C False** Osteitis is a medical emergency and antibiotic treatment must be initiated immediately on a 'best-guess' basis because of the risks of bone necrosis, septic arthritis, septicaemia and metastatic infection. Blood culture results may take 24 hours and should not be depended on to the extent of delaying treatment, although when sensitivities are available they may modify treatment.

**D  False**  Under the age of 5, a significant proportion of acute osteitis is caused by *Haemophilus influenzae* and antibiotic therapy should cover both this organism and the far more common *Staphylococcus pyogenes*. Either amoxycillin or a third generation cephalosporin should be used in combination with flucloxacillin. Over the age of 5, *Staphylococcus pyogenes* dominates to such an extent that a combination of either benzylpenicillin and cloxacillin, or cloxacillin and sodium fusidate is appropriate first choice treatment pending sensitivities. All antibiotics given should be in high dosage and by the intravenous route. *Haemophilous* osteitis has a characteristic tendency to cause apparent bruising over the lesion, to such an extent that cases of maxillary osteitis have been regarded as due to non-accidental injury.

**E  True**  Acute lymphatic leukaemia may present as bone pain. If this is the diagnosis, X-rays will usually show bony rarefaction. A normal peripheral blood film would not exclude leukaemia in this situation, and bone marrow biopsy would be indicated.

**F2  A  False**  'Dextrose saline' is a quite unsuitable fluid for the treatment of shock. Plasma is the treatment of choice in a dose of 20 ml/kg given rapidly and repeated if necessary; 0.9% saline should be used while plasma is being obtained.

**B  False**  This condition is so clinically distinct and can cause such rapid deterioration that treatment may be granted precedence over investigation. Thus it is entirely appropriate for a family doctor to inject benzylpenicillin prior to sending a child into hospital, and for a hospital doctor to do the same, if there is any difficulty or delay in obtaining blood or CSF. Even after prior penicillin there is a good chance of culturing the meningococcus from a throat swab. Gram stain of fluid from a skin lesion can also be diagnostic.

**C  True**  The formula of 20 ml/kg is derived from this on the grounds that in shock the vascular compartment is likely to be at least 25% depleted.

**D  True**  The meningitis is very responsive to treatment. It is septicaemia complicated by disseminated intravascular coagulation that is the main cause of mortality.

**E** **False** Shock may be defined as a state where the circulation is insufficient to meet tissue requirements. Cold peripheries, poor venous filling and poor capillary return are all good evidence for shock. The blood pressure may be maintained until very late in shock due to maximal vasoconstriction, and 'shock' should be diagnosed and treated before this late stage.

**F3** **A** **True** Fractures crossing any of the sinuses, or involving the middle ear or mastoid air cells, can predispose to cerebral abscess formation by allowing bacteria access to brain tissue.

**B** **True** Pyogenic lung abscess or bronchiectasis can predispose to cerebral abscess formation because bacteria can bypass the normal filtering action of the lungs by draining via the pulmonary veins to the left side of the heart and thence to cerebral vessels.

**C** **False**

**D** **False** Only right-to-left shunts predispose to cerebral abscess formation. They enable bacteria from areas of peripheral sepsis (e.g. boils) to enter the cerebral circulation having bypassed the filtering action of the lungs.

**E** **True**

**F4** **A** **False** Vasoconstriction precedes vasodilatation. Both intra-and extracranial vessels may be affected, so that in the prodromal phase vasoconstriction may manifest itself respectively as hemiplegia/hemianaesthesia and facial pallor. The subsequent vasodilatation gives migraine headache its characteristic throbbing character.

**B** **True** Vasoconstriction of branches of the middle cerebral artery may cause ischaemia to portions of the optic radiation resulting in homonymous hemianopia.

**C** **True** Recurrent abdominal pains are commonly ascribed to 'abdominal migraine'. Like classic migraine they tend to be paroxysmal and potentially severe with intervening periods of normal health. As the child grows older, headaches may begin to feature more prominently in attacks until they eventually replace the abdominal pain.

**D** **False** Ergotamine is a vasoconstrictor drug, and as vasoconstriction is the basis of migrainous hemiplegia ergotamine is contraindicated in this variety of migraine.

**E** **False** In both adolescent girls and adult women migraine is characteristically either premenstrual in timing or during a period.

**F5** **A** **False** Meconium aspiration pneumonia is very much a disease of *term* infants, who are especially liable to both pass and inhale meconium if subjected to intrapartum asphyxia. Once meconium-containing liquor enters the respiratory tract it causes a chemical pneumonitis with airways obstruction. There are areas of both collapse and overinflation with a high risk of pneumothorax.

**B** **True** Infants with L:S ratios of greater than 2:1 virtually never develop hyaline membrane disease, as such a ratio is evidence that surfactant is present in abundance in the infant's lungs. Some infants with ratios of between 1.5:1 and 2:1 develop HMD, and 70% of those with ratios less than 1.5:1 do so. Good resuscitation with the avoidance of significant hypoxia, acidosis or hypothermia reduces the chance of an individual infant developing HMD; these insults can all lead to the destruction of surfactant already present.

**C** **False** The chest X-ray in HMD is typically 'ground glass' opacity with an air bronchogram. Patchy opacities favour an alternative diagnosis such as meconium aspiration pneumonia or a bacterial bronchopneumonia.

**D** **False** It is generally accepted that one of the main aetiological factors in bronchopulmonary dysplasia is high inspiratory pressures used in intermittent positive pressure ventilation (IPPV). Accordingly, high pressures (30 cm of water and above) are to be avoided if possible. However, certain situations warrant an increase in pressure to levels of 30–35 cm of water, e.g. in the early stages of IPPV in a case of severe HMD where lower pressures fail to prevent hypoxia and acidosis despite inspired oxygen concentrations of 95%. A short period of high pressure IPPV may serve to open up collapsed alveoli, allowing a return to lower pressures after several hours.

**E  False**    CPAP is not an effective management for a pneumothorax, and indeed pneumothorax is actually a complication of CPAP. All tension pneumothoraces should be drained urgently. Mature infants who are well and in whom the pneumothorax is small and not under tension can be treated conservatively.

**F6  A  False**    Prolonged convulsions should be aborted either by intravenous phenobarbitone or by intravenous or rectal diazepam. Thereafter phenobarbitone is probably the drug of first choice for maintenance therapy.

**B  True**    When other common causes of neonatal convulsions have been excluded (e.g. hypoglycaemia, hypocalcaemia, meningitis, etc.) a therapeutic trial of pyridoxine (vitamin $B_6$) should be administered in case the cause is 'pyridoxine dependency'.

**C  True**    Convulsive episodes may present as apnoeic attacks, especially in preterm infants. It is important to differentiate the two conditions as the management is different.

**D  False**    The majority of cases of neonatal convulsions end up being labelled idiopathic. A further proportion are due to relatively brief treatable conditions such as hypoglycaemia and hypocalcaemia. Overall, the prognosis for normal development in these groups is good.

**E  True**    The infant whose mother is a narcotic addict will suffer withdrawal symptoms at about 24 hours of age. The infant is likely to be irritable and sweaty and may have a tremor. Convulsions may result and should be controlled by anticonvulsants. It would seem reasonable to prescribe a narcotic for the infant in the short term and then wean him/her off over a few weeks. Use of naloxone at birth will precipitate even earlier withdrawal symptoms.

**F7  A  False**    A venous hum is usually heard in the erect position and should be abolished by lying the child flat or compressing the neck veins while auscultating.

**B   True**   At birth the pressure on the right side of the heart remains high comparable to that on the left. Accordingly, with a ventricular septal defect, left-to-right flow may be minimal and murmurs may not be present. The pulmonary vascular resistance falls over the first week of life leading to increased left-to-right flow and the appearance of the murmur. The 6-week baby check is a valuable opportunity to make good this potential defect in neonatal screening.

**C   True**   Significant left-to-right shunting causes an increase in the work of breathing due to 'stiff lungs'. This may be reflected in visible intercostal recession.

**D   False**   Normal femoral pulses at birth may occur despite severe preductal coarctation of the aorta, due to blood bypassing the obstruction via the patent ductus. The latter commonly closes in the first week of life leading to rapidly progressive heart failure. Treatment in the situation consists of the use of prostaglandins to keep the duct open and other supportive measures pending emergency surgery.

**E   False**   Peripheral oedema is often absent in cases of heart failure in infancy and childhood, and hepatomegaly is a far more reliable and valuable sign.

**F8   A   False**   Beclomethasone is an extremely effective and valuable drug in the long-term management of asthma. However, it is no substitute for systemic steroids in an acute attack.

**B   True**   The failure to respond to bronchodilators may be due to mucosal oedema and plugging. Early recourse to steroids is justifiable in view of their delayed mode of action, and such a policy may be expected to prevent deterioration and to shorten the attack.

**C   False**   Ketotifen has no place in the management of acute attacks of asthma. Its precise place in the long-term management of asthma remains a matter of some uncertainty.

**D   False**   Propranolol is a β blocker, and as such is positively contraindicated in any patient with asthma, as it could cause life-threatening deterioration.

**E**  **True**  In severe acute asthma, mucus plugging may render nebulized $\beta_2$ agonist therapy ineffective, and either parenteral $\beta_2$ agonists or aminophylline are indicated. Aminophylline remains a safe, effective and orthodox drug to use in the management of acute attacks of asthma, and acts synergically with $\beta$ agonists such as salbutamol. It should be administered slowly (over 5–15 minutes) and care should be taken to reduce dosage if there has been previous oral therapy with theophylline.

**F9**  **A**  **True**  Crohn's disease may present with vague malaise, pyrexia, recurrent abdominal pain or failure to thrive. If possible the diagnosis should be made by histology, e.g. from a rectal or colonoscopic biopsy, appendicectomy (occasionally) or at laparotomy leading to intestinal resection. Diagnosis may depend upon radiological features. Perianal lesions or abdominal masses are highly suggestive. Arthritis, clubbing, erythema nodosum and aphthous stomatitis are recognized associations. Mesenteric tuberculosis may give a very similar clinical and radiological picture and needs to be excluded in every case.

**B**  **False**  See (A).

**C**  **True**  See (A).

**D**  **True**  See (A).

**E**  **True**  See (A).

**F10**  **A**  **True**  Every child with cirrhosis should be investigated for Wilson's disease (hepatolenticular degeneration), as this is one of the few treatable causes of cirrhosis. Slit-lamp examination of the eyes may reveal Kayser–Fleischer rings which are pathognomonic of this condition; their absence does not exclude the diagnosis. Serum copper and caeruloplasmin are low, and treatment is with penicillamine.

**B**  **False**  Glycosylated haemoglobin is a useful test for assessing long-term diabetic control. It has no obvious value in the investigation of cirrhosis.

**C**  **True**  Congenital $\alpha_1$-antitrypsin deficiency is a rare cause of childhood cirrhosis, and is associated with emphysema in young adults. There is no definitive treatment for either condition.

**D   True**   Testing for reducing substances will be positive in galactosaemia. This condition usually presents in infancy with fulminating hepatic failure which may be fatal. However, some milder cases present in later childhood with cirrhosis and cataracts. Treatment is by a galactose-free diet.

**E   True**   While most cases of cystic fibrosis are usually diagnosed as a result of failure to thrive and recurrent chest infections, this condition does cause biliary cirrhosis and it is possible that mild cases might present in this way.

**F11   A   False**   Most cases of congenital adrenal hyperplasia will present in infancy and grow normally following treatment. Milder or incorrectly treated cases will show virilization, accelerated linear growth and precocious puberty. They will be taller than average prepubertally but early fusion of epiphyses will reduce the final adult height.

**B   True**   Crohn's disease can cause stunting of growth directly by causing malabsorption if it affects sufficient length of small intestine. In addition, it is a chronic inflammatory disease and most such diseases can have a deleterious effect on growth.

**C   False**   Boys with XXY karyotype (Klinefelter syndrome) are typically of average or above average height and suffer from hypogonadism.

**D   True**   Emotional deprivation is almost certainly the commonest cause of significant growth retardation, being much commoner than growth hormone deficiency. It is probably considerably underdiagnosed because affected children come from the type of families which cooperate poorly with medical investigation. In addition, short stature is often wrongly regarded as familial because the parents are also small, whereas they also may have suffered childhood deprivation. The definitive investigation in a suspected case is a therapeutic trial of an improved environment.

**E   True**   An XO karyotype (Turner syndrome) occurs in about 1:3000 live births, and affected girls are usually significantly short from early childhood.

**F12**  **A**  **False**  *Pneumocystis carinii* is a protozoan of low pathogenicity which is recognized as a significant threat to the immunologically compromised population of children with leukaemia. It causes a characteristic chest X-ray consisting of diffuse ground glass infiltration. Confirmation of the diagnosis during life may be difficult and a therapeutic trial of drug treatment is justifiable on clinical suspicion. Pentamidine was formerly the drug of choice but has been superseded by high-dose cotrimoxazole (20 mg/kg/day). Erythromycin is not effective.

  **B**  **True**  This is because it is a live virus that could behave with increased virulence in an immunocompromised host. If a child with leukaemia is exposed to measles he/she should be given passive protection with pooled gammaglobulin.

  **C**  **True**  Cranial irradiation is routine as prophylaxis against meningeal relapse. Growth hormone deficiency has occurred as a result.

  **D**  **False**  Although the population of long-term female survivors of childbearing age is small, some have already given birth to normal children.

  **E**  **False**  Allopurinol is indicated only in the first induction phase when the leukaemic cell mass is very large.

**F13**  **A**  **False**  Spherocytosis occurs commonly in ABO incompatibility, which will be included in the differential diagnosis of neonates with haemolytic jaundice.

  **B**  **True**

  **C**  **False**  The Coombs' test will be negative in every case, as the haemolysis in this condition has nothing to do with autoimmunity; the haemolysis in spherocytosis occurs because of the intrinsic defect in the red cell which leads to a shortened life span and increased destruction in the spleen.

  **D**  **True**  Spherocytosis causes neonatal jaundice with a significant frequency, and sometimes the jaundice is severe enough to need exchange transfusion.

    **E**   **False**   Splenectomy *is* the treatment for the more severe varieties of this condition and it will invariably cure the anaemia, abolish the jaundice and reticulocytosis and return the red cell survival time to near normal. However, it does nothing for the intrinsic defect in the red cell, so spherocytosis persists. The optimal age for splenectomy remains a matter for debate because of the resultant impaired immunity. The child should receive pneumococcal vaccination prior to splenectomy and thereafter receive prophylactic penicillin, probably for life.

**F14**  **A**  **True**   Posterior urethral valves are a congenital form of obstruction to bladder emptying. The bladder becomes enlarged and back pressure may cause hydronephrosis with renal damage which may occur to a significant extent *in utero*. The bladder empties by dribbling overflow and may be palpable. Cases have been detected antenatally by ultrasound scan which allows early treatment in the neonatal period. Treatment consists of diathermy to the valves.

    **B**   **False**   Whereas previously circumcision has been performed for non-retractility of the prepuce under the age of 3–5 years, it is now recognized that most non-retractile prepuces will become retractile if left alone. 8% of 6-year olds have a non-retractile prepuce, but this declines to 1% at 16 years.

    **C**   **False**   Up to 5% of children still wet the bed at 10 years of age. This does not mean that they should be regarded as normal, as it is an unpleasant and embarrassing problem for child and family alike and is amenable to treatment. A very small minority of cases may be due to an organic problem. In the majority of the remainder some environmental or psychological problem will have interfered with the acquisition of bladder control at the critical period for this skill, viz. between the ages of 2–4 years.

    **D**   **True**   Marked vesicoureteric reflux leads to incomplete voiding of a full bladder because a significant proportion of the urine flows back into the dilated ureters. This portion returns to the bladder sometimes leaving a sufficient volume to lead to a further desire to micturate. Double micturition is both a symptom and a treatment for vesicoureteric reflux.

E   **False**   The significant level is over 100 000 organisms per ml. This is for a single organism and assuming clean collection of a fresh urine. Mixed growths are suggestive of contamination.

**F15**   A   **True**   It is likely that the high level of secretory IgA in breast milk is one of the factors responsible for the lower incidence of gastroenteritis in breast fed infants. It may also have a role in protecting the infant's immune system from foreign proteins entering the gut.

B   **True**   Breast milk contains lactose as its main source of carbohydrate. This is split by digestion to glucose and galactose, and the latter is toxic in infants with galactosaemia. The latter condition is therefore one of the few genuine contraindications to breast feeding.

C   **False**   Breast milk does not contain fructose, which is most likely to be encountered by an infant when sucrose (as table sugar) is added to a bottle, or when fruit juice is first given. (Both are common practices in the treatment of constipation.)

D   **True**   Prolactin (from the anterior pituitary) is important both for initiating milk production before birth and for maintaining its production after birth. Suckling stimulates both prolactin and oxytocin release. The latter stimulates the 'let-down' reflex.

E   **True**   Breast milk contains both less phosphorus and less calcium than cow's milk. The high phosphorus content of cow's milk was associated with 'cow's milk tetany', and idiopathic hypercalcaemia is virtually unknown in breast fed infants.

**F16**   A   **True**   The limbs are short relative to the trunk thus resembling an old looking 2-year-old child. This condition in its full-blown form is due to severe emotional and nutritional deprivation. Growth stunting may be severe with near total growth arrest and retarded bone age. Catch-up growth on removal to a more nurturing environment may be dramatic.

B   **True**   The mechanism whereby emotional deprivation causes a pot belly is not fully understood. Its presence may mask the overall poor nutritional state of the child. The pot belly disappears in response to an improvement of the child's environment.

**C  False**  Marked psychomotor retardation in all fields is common, especially with regard to speech and language. This is probably due to understimulation and simple lack of exposure to language. All areas of development show catch-up in response to an improved environment, but speech is understandably one of the areas in which improvements are slowest.

**D  False**  Normal parents would be very reluctant to leave a 4-year-old child alone in hospital, and a normal 4-year-old child would object strongly to such a course of action. In contrast, parents of 'deprivation dwarfs' are usually quite happy to leave their children in hospital and visit infrequently. The child characteristically is perfectly happy with the arrangement and improves dramatically in the hospital setting, showing far more interest in the hospital staff than in his parents. The situation is complicated by the fact that milder cases of the syndrome may show exaggerated 'anxious attachment' to their parent figures.

**E  True**  This is one of the hallmarks of deprived children. They both show and demand affectionate interaction with every stranger with whom they come into contact. Although they may develop favourites, their behaviour is essentially promiscuous.

**F17  A  True**  The mean age to acquire this skill is 6 months and delay beyond the age of 9 months should be regarded as abnormal.

**B  False**  25% of normal children may be unable to stand unaided by their first birthday.

**C  True**  The upper limit of normal for sitting without support is at about 8 months.

**D  False**  This is entirely within normal limits.

**E  True**  A normal 1-year-old baby should show strong attachment behaviour to his mother and be unable to tolerate admission to hospital without protest. Easy acceptance of separation by both mother and child is a serious reflection on the mother–child relationship and on the quality of the previous care-giving.

**F18  A  True**   Most cases of ovarian dysgenesis have a 45 XO chromosome pattern giving a chromatin negative buccal smear. However, a small number of cases have normal chromosomes despite having the phenotype of Turner syndrome. The practical value of the buccal smear examination is that it can give an answer several days earlier than chromosome examination which is obviously of value in the neonatal period.

**B  False**   Clitoral hypertrophy is not a feature of Turner syndrome as there is no reason for any increase in androgenic activity. Clitoral hypertrophy in a newborn female is usually due to congenital adrenal hyperplasia.

**C  True**   Oedema of the hands and feet in the neonatal period is a characteristic finding in Turner syndrome, although its cause is unknown. Other features include webbing of the neck, a redundant fold of skin on the back of the neck, cubitus valgus, and a broad 'shieldshaped' chest with widely spaced nipples. In later childhood short stature, primary amenorrhoea and lack of secondary sex characteristics at the age of puberty are to be expected.

**D  False**   Syndactyly is not connected with Turner syndrome being an isolated condition which is usually inherited as an autosomal dominant. (Abnormalities of the fingernails have been described in Turner syndrome; namely increased transverse curvature of the nails.)

**E  True**   Associated congenital heart disease is the main serious medical complication of Turner syndrome, the commonest variety being coarctation of the aorta. This contrasts with the situation in Noonan syndrome (male Turner syndrome, Bonnevie–Ulrich syndrome) in which similar bodily features occur in male infants with undescended tests and normal chromosomes; the heart defect most commonly found in this condition is pulmonary stenosis.

**F19  A  True**   Medulloblastoma is the commonest tumour of the central nervous system in childhood. It commonly arises from the vermis of the cerebellum and presents either as cerebellar ataxia, raised intracranial pressure or both.

**B   False**   Meningioma of the falx cerebri has no effect on cerebellar function. It is most likely to cause a spastic paraplegia by virtue of its strategic position close to the areas of motor cortex supplying both legs.

**C   False**   Polio only affects lower motor neurons and so does not cause cerebellar signs.

**D   True**   Varicella encephalitis has a predilection for the cerebellum. It is usually a mild and self-limiting disease.

**E   False**   Dystonia musculorum deformans is a rare condition affecting the extrapyramidal system but not the cerebellum. Bizarre postures of one or other limb are common, and because of its rarity cases are usually regarded as hysterical in origin for months or years.

**F20   A   True**   A lesion placed centrally in the cervical cord will affect spinothalamic fibres as they cross the midline to reach the lateral spinothalamic tracts, but tend to spare fibres which ascend uncrossed in the posterior columns. This will result in 'dissociated anaesthesia' i.e. loss of pain and temperature sensation with preservation of proprioception, vibration sense and deep pain sensation. This will tend to occur in a 'cape-like' distribution over the arms and shoulders, depending on the vertical extent of the lesion.

**B   True**   An intrinsic lesion of the cervical cord is very likely to cause Horner syndrome by damaging the sympathetic tract just lateral to the grey matter. Horner syndrome consists of ptosis and enophthalmos, together with a constricted pupil (the latter caused by overaction of the parasympathetic fibres). In addition there is loss of sweating over the affected side of the face.

**C   False**   Any leg involvement secondary to a cervical cord lesion must be an upper motor neuron lesion, in which there may be weakness but there will be no wasting.

**D   False**   A cervical cord lesion cannot cause nystagmus, which can only be due to cerebellar, brain stem or vestibular involvement, or else ocular in origin.

**E   True**   The sensory portion of the Vth cranial nerve has a tract which descends into the cervical cord. Accordingly, sensory loss in the trigeminal area can result from cervical cord lesions.

# PAPER G
## QUESTIONS

**G1** **The following conditions cause a hypokalaemic alkalosis:**
- A haemolytic uraemic syndrome.
- B infantile hypertrophic pyloric stenosis.
- C diabetic ketosis.
- D Bartter syndrome.
- E steroid therapy.

**G2** **In the acutely dyspnoeic 2-year-old child:**
- A respiratory difficulty on inspiration localizes obstruction to the lower bronchial tree.
- B the presence of dysphagia and drooling of saliva suggests that *Haemophilus influenzae* is a likely causative organism.
- C asthma is an unlikely diagnosis at this age.
- D if the blood gases are normal this makes the diagnosis of laryngeal obstruction very unlikely.
- E if chest X-ray shows multiple small fluid levels, the causative organism is likely to be *Mycoplasma pneumoniae*.

**G3** **The following conditions may result in total villous atrophy of the small bowel mucosa:**
- A *Giardia lamblia* infection.
- B cow's milk protein intolerance.
- C viral gastroenteritis.
- D cystic fibrosis.
- E congenital lactose intolerance.

**G4** **The following are recognized causes of macroglossia in infancy:**
- A spinal muscular atrophy Type I.
- B rhabdomyosarcoma.
- C Type II glycogen storage disease.
- D Hurler syndrome (gargoylism).
- E hepatolenticular degeneration.

**G5** **The following statements are correct:**
- A hypermetropia may cause a convergent strabismus.
- B hereditary fructose intolerance may cause cataracts.
- C retrolental fibroplasia may lead to retinal detachment.

    **D**   systemic corticosteroids may cause cataracts if administered for over a year.

    **E**   dislocation of the lens may occur in homocystinuria.

**G6**    **The incubation periods for the following infectious fevers are:**
    **A**   rubella: 7–10 days.
    **B**   measles: 10–14 days.
    **C**   varicella: 21 days.
    **D**   mumps: 7–10 days.
    **E**   pertussis: 7 days.

**G7**    **The fetal alcohol syndrome is characterized by:**
    **A**   a single palmar crease.
    **B**   maxillary hypoplasia.
    **C**   excess lanugo.
    **D**   psychomotor retardation.
    **E**   increased birth weight.

**G8**    **The following statements concerning measles are correct:**
    **A**   immunization is maximally effective if given at 6 months of age.
    **B**   the rash appears on the second day of the illness.
    **C**   the risk of developing subacute sclerosing panencephalitis (SSPE) is about 1 in 10 000 cases.
    **D**   the incubation period is from 15–21 days.
    **E**   immunization is contraindicated in children with cystic fibrosis.

**G9**    **In respiratory distress syndrome (RDS) due to meconium aspiration:**
    **A**   antibiotic therapy is of crucial importance.
    **B**   steroid therapy improves the prognosis.
    **C**   there is a high risk of pneumothorax.
    **D**   chest X-ray typically shows 'ground glass' opacity.
    **E**   the infant may also suffer from cerebral oedema.

**G10**    **Recognized associations of 'small-for-dates' babies include:**
    **A**   maternal smoking in pregnancy.
    **B**   haemolytic disease due to ABO incompatibility.
    **C**   pre-eclamptic toxaemia.
    **D**   congenital rubella infection.
    **E**   fetal alcohol syndrome.

**G11**    **In atrial septal defect (ASD):**
    **A**   left axis deviation on ECG suggests ostium primum defect.
    **B**   the characteristic murmur is due to flow across the septal defect.
    **C**   there may be an associated diastolic murmur in the mitral area.

D ostium secundum defects are associated with mitral incompetence.
E the pulmonary component of the second sound is diminished in intensity.

**G12 The following may occur in craniopharyngioma:**
A punched-out radiolucent areas on skull X-ray.
B homonymous hemianopia.
C increased sensitivity to insulin.
D polyuria.
E retarded bone age.

**G13 In idiopathic thrombocytopenic purpura (ITP):**
A the purpuric rash is characteristically on the buttocks and the extensor surfaces of the limbs.
B bone marrow examination characteristically reveals diminished numbers of megakaryocytes.
C the infant of an affected mother may develop transient thrombocytopenia.
D steroid therapy is ineffective.
E the prothrombin time is prolonged.

**G14 In von Recklinghausen's disease (neurofibromatosis):**
A as few as three café-au-lait spots are diagnostic.
B axillary freckling supports the diagnosis.
C there is a recognized association with scoliosis.
D there is an autosomal recessive form of inheritance.
E fibromas usually only appear at puberty.

**G15 The following statements concerning juvenile rheumatoid arthritis (Still's disease) are correct:**
A rheumatoid factor is usually positive.
B pericarditis is a recognized feature.
C a recognized presentation is with a pyrexia persisting for up to several months.
D the typical pattern of joint involvement differs from that in Henoch–Schönlein syndrome.
E subcutaneous nodules may occur.

**G16 The following are characteristic features of rickets:**
A decreased bone density on X-ray.
B normal or low alkaline phosphatase.
C widening and 'fraying' of epiphyses on X-ray.
D raised serum phosphate.
E subperiosteal new bone formation.

**G17 In a 7-year-old child who presents with soiling:**
A a history of deposition of formed stool behind the settee is an indication to proceed to a barium enema.

**B**  rectal examination may be justified.
**C**  hospital admission should only be considered as a last resort.
**D**  there is more than a 50% chance that the diagnosis is Hirschsprung's disease.
**E**  if the soiling consists of the frequent involuntary passage of small quantities of stool, this suggests the problem is psychological in origin.

**G18**  **The following are characteristic features of dermatomyositis in childhood:**
   **A**  calcification of skin lesions.
   **B**  pericarditis.
   **C**  hypercalcaemia.
   **D**  tenderness and weakness of limb girdle muscles.
   **E**  muscle biopsy is diagnostic.

**G19**  **The following conditions cause nystagmus:**
   **A**  basilar artery migraine.
   **B**  Friedreich's ataxia.
   **C**  phenytoin toxicity.
   **D**  congenital cataract.
   **E**  Guillain–Barré syndrome.

**G20**  **In the management of childhood epilepsy:**
   **A**  swimming should be prohibited.
   **B**  phenobarbitone may cause gum hyperplasia.
   **C**  infantile spasms may respond to ACTH.
   **D**  most patients should be educated in special schools.
   **E**  anticonvulsant medication should be prescribed for 2–3 years after a first non-febrile convulsion.

# PAPER G
## ANSWERS

**G1**  **A**  **False**   Haemolytic uraemic syndrome is a condition which can lead to acute renal failure. The vast majority of cases are associated with a severe diarrhoeal illness caused by a verotoxin-producing strain of *E. coli* (usually 0157). The renal failure is associated with microangiopathic haemolytic anaemia and thrombocytopenia and causes *acidosis* with hyperkalaemia for which dialysis is often required.

     **B**  **True**   Infants with pyloric stenosis suffer repeated vomiting with loss of $H^+$ ions and $K^+$ ions, which leads to a metabolic alkalosis with hypokalaemia. A period of intravenous fluid therapy with potassium replacement is indicated preoperatively in infants where these derangements are significant.

     **C**  **False**   In diabetic ketosis there is *acidosis* because of accumulation of keto acids. Although total body potassium is usually considerably depleted, the serum potassium before treatment is usually elevated as a result of intracellular potassium being displaced by $H^+$ ions to compensate for the acidosis in the extracellular fluid. This initial high serum potassium should not prevent early potassium supplementation after the initial 1–4-hour period of rapid extracellular fluid replacement.

     **D**  **True**   Bartter syndrome is a rare condition, inherited as an autosomal recessive, which is thought to be due to vascular unresponsiveness to angiotensin. This leads to hypertrophy of the juxtaglomerular apparatus (which can be detected by renal biopsy) with increased renin secretion. This leads to angiotensin release and secondary hyperaldosteronism. The resultant hypokalaemic alkalosis is a hallmark of the condition, which usually presents as unexplained failure to thrive. Polyuria and polydipsia are usually present together with constipation and muscle weakness.

**E** **True**   Both hydrocortisone and synthetic steroids such as prednisolone act on the distal renal tubule to cause sodium retention and potassium excretion with resultant hypokalaemia. As with most causes of hypokalaemia there is an associated metabolic alkalosis due to renal attempts to conserve potassium at the expense of hydrogen ions.

**G2** **A** **False**   Inspiratory difficulty is characteristic of laryngeal obstruction or obstruction in the immediate subglottic area. Obstruction to the lower bronchial tree (as in asthma) is typically worse on expiration.

**B** **True**   Dysphagia and drooling are both suggestive of acute epiglottitis due to *Haemophilus influenzae*. This condition should become increasingly rare as a result of the routine incorporation of Hib vaccine into immunization schedules.

**C** **False**   The majority of cases of severe asthma have attacks which start in the first year of life, and while at this age it may be difficult to differentiate any one attack from bronchiolitis, it is advisable both to diagnose and treat acute wheeze in the second year of life as asthma until proved otherwise.

**D** **False**   A child with moderate laryngeal obstruction can compensate for the obstruction by increased respiratory effort. Blood gases usually remain normal until very late, when increasing obstruction can cause rapid deterioration.

**E** **False**   The causative organism will usually be *Staphylococcus pyogenes*. *Mycoplasma pneumoniae* does not cause destruction of lung tissue or abscess formation, but instead causes a patchy interstitial pneumonitis in the lower lobes.

**G3** **A** **False**   *Giardia lamblia* can cause steatorrhoea and the malabsorption syndrome or be totally asymptomatic. Absence of cystic or free forms in the stool does not exclude the diagnosis. Jejunal biopsy can confirm the diagnosis. Giardiasis sometimes causes partial villous atrophy. Treatment consists of a course of oral metronidazole.

**B** **True**   Cow's milk protein intolerance can cause a wide variety of symptoms, including diarrhoea, vomiting, colic, rectal bleeding and failure to thrive. Intolerance can be primary or else secondary to viral gastroenteritis. The severest cases may have total villous atrophy. Treatment is by exclusion of cow's milk protein from the diet.

**C** **True** A severe episode of viral gastroenteritis can cause total villous atrophy.

**D** **False** The small bowel is normal in cystic fibrosis, and the failure to thrive in this condition is secondary to digestive failure (due to pancreatic insufficiency), not absorptive failure.

**E** **False** Congenital lactose intolerance is a rare condition in which the small intestinal morphology is normal but the enzyme lactase is deficient. Secondary lactose intolerance may exist in conditions causing total villous atrophy such as coeliac disease and gastroenteritis; however, it does not in itself cause villous atrophy.

**G4** **A** **False** Type I spinal muscular atrophy (Werdnig–Hoffmann disease) does not cause macroglossia. Being a disease characterized by degeneration of lower motor neurons it causes weakness and wasting of all skeletal muscles, including the tongue. Fasciculation of tongue muscles is one of the cardinal signs of the disease. The disease is inherited as an autosomal recessive, and causes death usually by the first birthday.

**B** **True** Rhabdomyosarcoma is a rare but highly malignant tumour which arises from smooth muscle fibres, and can occur virtually anywhere in the body, including the tongue. It is probably the commonest neoplastic cause of macroglossia.

**C** **True** Type II glycogen storage disease (Pompe's disease) is characterized by glycogen deposition in liver and muscle. This results in both macroglossia and cardiomyopathy, the latter resulting in cardiac failure in early infancy.

**D** **True** Hurler syndrome (gargoylism) is a mucopolysaccharidosis which, in addition to macroglossia, is characterized by coarse facies, severe retardation, clouding of the cornea and hepatosplenomegaly. Lateral spine X-ray shows a characteristic beak-shaped deformity of several vertebral bodies. Diagnosis can be confirmed by finding dermatan and heparan sulphate in the urine. Inheritance is usually as an autosomal recessive. Recently there have been encouraging reports of treatment by marrow transplantation.

**E   False**   Hepatolenticular degeneration (Wilson's disease) is a condition inherited as an autosomal recessive characterized by deposition of copper in the brain, liver and kidneys. This results respectively in extrapyramidal signs, cirrhosis and renal tubular damage. There are low serum levels of both copper and caeruloplasmin, and slit-lamp examination of the cornea reveals the diagnostic Kayser–Fleischer rings. This condition should be considered in *all* children with liver disease, and when found should lead to screening of siblings. The condition does not cause macroglossia.

**G5   A   True**   Conversely, myopia leads to underconvergence and a divergent strabismus.

**B   False**   There is a disorder of monosaccharide metabolism which causes cataract, namely galactosaemia.

**C   True**   In retrolental fibroplasia retinal vessels proliferate and grow forward into the vitreous. Later stages include vitreous haemorrhage with fibrosis leading to retinal detachment.

**D   True**   The children most likely to need such therapy are those with steroid-dependent nephrotic syndrome or severe asthma.

**E   True**   This also occurs in the clinically very similar condition of Marfan syndrome.

**G6   A   False**   14–21 days.

**B   True**

**C   False**   1–14 days.

**D   False**   16–21 days.

**E   True**

**G7   A   False**

**B   True**   This condition consists of microcephaly, abnormal facies, low birth weight and global retardation which may be severe. The extent to which milder versions of the syndrome are being missed is of some interest.

**C   False**

**D   True**   See (A).

**E   False**   See (A).

**G8 A False** Measles vaccine is a live vaccine, and is less likely to 'take' if administered in the first 6 months of life because of passive immunity from the mother. The susceptibility to both the illness and the vaccine increases after the age of 6 months, and is maximal in the second year of life. In the UK, the vaccine is offered shortly after the first birthday. In developing countries vaccine should be given between 9 and 10 months of age because children develop measles much younger and it is a far more serious disease.

**B False** The rash appears on the fourth day of the illness. This leads to the common event of a child admitted to hospital (for example, because of a febrile convulsion) coming out in a measles rash just before the consultant's ward round! The only way measles can be diagnosed before the rash appears is by seeing Koplik's spots which usually occur on the second day of the illness.

**C False** The risk is about 1 in 100 000. The risk of 'ordinary' measles encephalitis is around 1 in 1000–5000 and the possible sequelae of the condition are the main reason for the measles vaccination campaign.

**D False** The incubation period of measles is 10–14 days.

**E False** Children with cystic fibrosis deserve protection from measles even more than normal children, because they would be especially prone to the respiratory complications of measles, especially the secondary bacterial bronchopneumonia.

**G9 A False** Some units do use antibiotics in meconium aspiration pneumonia but it is quite respectable to withhold them. Meconium itself is sterile.

**B False** Steroid therapy has no effect on the course of the disease in meconium aspiration pneumonia.

**C True** Pneumothorax is a common complication of meconium aspiration syndrome as is pneumomediastinum. It results from the tendency to air trapping and over-distension of areas of lung which is characteristic of this condition.

**D False** A chest X-ray showing ground glass opacity is typical of hyaline membrane disease. The X-ray in meconium aspiration shows patchy areas of atelectasis and air trapping with an overall tendency to hyperinflation.

**E    True**    Meconium aspiration occurs in the context of severe intrapartum asphyxia. This asphyxia is likely to result in cerebral hypoxia, which may in turn result in significant cerebral oedema. This latter complication may be aggravated by inappropriate ADH secretion which also commonly occurs as a result of cerebral hypoxia.

**G10   A    True**    Maternal smoking in pregnancy is significantly associated with low birth weight infants. The mechanism is thought to be partially due to reduced placental blood flow. It has been roughly estimated that smoking 20 cigarettes a day can reduce the infant's birth weight by 0.5 kg. It seems likely that some of the excess perinatal mortality observed in social classes IV and V is related to the greater tendency to smoking in pregnancy in these population groups.

**B    False**    ABO incompatibility is due to the development of anti-A or anti-B haemolysins in the mother of a baby who is A or B respectively. These haemolysins are IgG antibodies and cross the placenta. However, the A and B antigens only develop on fetal red cells during the last 4 weeks of pregnancy so the process (which is anyway much less severe than haemolytic disease due to Rhesus isoimmunization) does not affect fetal growth significantly. Infants with ABO incompatibility are usually well-grown, full-term specimens.

**C    True**    The precise aetiology of pre-eclampsia is still not fully understood, but a prominent feature of it is placental insufficiency and fetal growth retardation, leading to 'small-for-dates' infants.

**D    True**    Infants who have been affected by congenital rubella in the first trimester may have microcephaly, congenital heart disease and visual and auditory handicap. They are also usually 'small-for-dates'.

**E    True**    The fetal alcohol syndrome is characterized by abnormal facies, microcephaly and subsequent psychomotor retardation and low birth weight. Uncertainty exists as to the frequency of mild versions of this syndrome, and as to the quantity of alcohol ingestion needed to cause it. Infants of mothers who are true alcoholics are obviously at considerable risk.

**G11** **A** **True** The ECG in ostium primum defects characteristically shows both left axis deviation and incomplete right bundle branch block.

**B** **False** The flow across the defect is at low pressure through both systole and diastole and does not produce a murmur. The characteristic murmur of an ASD is an ejection murmur in the pulmonary area due to increased flow across the pulmonary valve. This murmur is very similar to that of pulmonary stenosis; the presence of a thrill would favour the latter.

**C** **False** There may be an additional soft *tricuspid* diastolic flow murmur in an ASD in which case this suggests that the degree of left-to-right shunting is significant enough to warrant further investigation. The analogous situation, in which there is a *mitral* diastolic flow murmur, is in ventricular septal defect.

**D** **False** Ostium primum defects are associated with mitral incompetence.

**E** **False** The pulmonary component of the second sound (P2) may be diminished in pulmonary valvar stenosis. In ASD, P2 will be normal or loud depending on the extent to which pulmonary hypertension has developed. There is widened 'fixed' splitting of the aortic and pulmonary components of the second sound.

**G12** **A** **False** Craniopharyngioma is a cause of intracranial calcification, not of radiolucency. The calcification is typically diffusely situated in the suprasellar region. The classic cause of punched-out lytic skull lesions is the histiocytosis X group of conditions.

**B** **False** A craniopharyngioma will tend to compress the optic chiasm, affecting crossing fibres from the nasal fields of each retina. It thus causes a bitemporal hemianopia. Homonymous hemianopia can only result from unilateral lesions of the optic pathways distal to the optic chiasm, i.e. of the optic tract, optic radiation or occipital cortex.

**C** **True** Craniopharyngioma commonly causes quite severe growth hormone deficiency, which leads to increased sensitivity to the hypoglycaemic effects of insulin. Thus, when growth hormone deficiency is being investigated by means of the insulin stress test, it is wise to use half the normal dose of insulin in a case of advanced craniopharyngioma.

**D  True**    Polyuria, polydipsia and nocturia may all occur in craniopharyngioma owing to involvement of the posterior pituitary causing diabetes insipidus.

**E  True**    Retarded bone age is likely in craniopharyngioma, secondary both to growth hormone deficiency and possibly to secondary hypothyroidism. Catch-up growth and return to normal bone age is likely with replacement therapy.

**G13  A  False**    The purpuric rash in ITP has no characteristic distribution. The distribution mentioned is typical of Henoch–Schönlein purpura.

**B  False**    The number of megakaryocytes is normal or increased with possible decreased budding, and otherwise normal findings.

**C  True**    This is probably due to transplacental passage of antiplatelet antibodies, and can occur after the mother has apparently been cured by splenectomy.

**D  False**    Steroid therapy is rapidly effective in the majority of cases for which it is prescribed. The indications are severe purpura and spontaneous bleeding from mucous membranes, with a platelet count below 20 000/mm$^3$. The aim of therapy is to prevent serious intracranial or other haemorrhage, of which there is a 1% risk. Immunoglobulin can be used instead of or in conjunction with steroids, and will probably raise the platelet count faster than steroids alone.

**E  False**    Thrombocytopenia leads to a prolonged bleeding time, and there is no reason for the prothrombin time to be prolonged as there is no abnormality of coagulation factors in ITP.

**G14  A  False**    A diagnosis of von Recklinghausen's disease rests on the clinical picture together with a positive family history. The tendency to develop café-au-lait spots increases with age and, although three spots in early childhood would be highly suggestive, the statement as it stands is incorrect and the diagnostic number usually accepted is five.

**B  True**    Axillary freckling is characteristic of neurofibromatosis and usually appears in early childhood. Its presence therefore strongly supports the diagnosis in a suspected case.

**C** **True** The association between scoliosis and neurofibromatosis is well recognized but unexplained as the scoliosis is not usually secondary to any specific features of the disease.

**D** **False** Von Recklinghausen's disease is inherited as an autosomal dominant and is a suitable condition for genetic counselling in view of its potentially unfortunate complications, which include mental defect, epilepsy, optic nerve gliomata and problems with nerve and spinal cord compression.

**E** **True** The skin fibromas which are characteristic of this condition do not usually appear until puberty.

**G15** **A** **False**

**B** **True**

**C** **True** There may be no clinical evidence of joint involvement during this period. There is often a polymorphic erythematous rash over the same period.

**D** **True** In Henoch–Schönlein syndrome large joints tend to be affected, often asymmetrically. In Still's disease both large and small joints are affected, usually symmetrically.

**E** **True** These occur over bony prominences and tendons and may be indistinguishable from those found in acute rheumatic fever.

**G16** **A** **True**

**B** **False** Alkaline phosphatase is always very high.

**C** **True** Together with the decreased bone density these X-ray findings are virtually pathognomonic of rickets.

**D** **False** Plasma phosphate tends to be low, due to increased urine loss secondary to increased parathyroid activity.

**E** **False** This is a feature of scurvy, or non-accidental injury, both of which cause subperiosteal haemorrhage which subsequently calcifies.

**G17** **A** **False** The typical 'psychological' soiler has an empty rectum, and passes formed stools in inappropriate places. Such children are not necessarily seriously disturbed, but certainly some of them may merit eventual referral to a child psychiatrist. There is no reason to consider an organic bowel disorder or to perform a barium enema in such cases.

**B   True**   Although some child psychiatrists regard rectal examination in such cases with disfavour, it is virtually essential to differentiate cases of constipation-with-overflow from those that are purely psychological in origin. In the former the severity of the impaction of faeces may be evaluated together with the possible need for an enema.

**C   False**   Whether the soiling is psychological or mechanical in origin, or a combination, early hospital admission may be very useful. In the psychological cases it breaks the parent-child interaction, and thus stops the soiling at least in the short term. In the management of constipation-with-overflow, it may facilitate the attainment of an empty rectum and then be useful in the relearning of a regular bowel pattern.

**D   False**   Hirschsprung's disease accounts for only a tiny fraction of all the cases of soiling in the childhood population.

**E   False**   This pattern is characteristic of constipation-with-overflow. Treatment with laxatives may result in an initial worsening of the soiling, but once the rectum is properly emptied the soiling should cease.

**G18   A   True**   Dermatomyositis is extremely rare in childhood and carries a poor prognosis. It presents insidiously with the triad of facial erythema, muscle weakness and fatigue. There are patches of erythema on knuckles, elbows and knees with a tendency to induration of subcutaneous tissues. The erythematous skin is said to have a violaceous or heliotrope colouration. Skin lesions may calcify and ulcerate.

**B   False**

**C   False**

**D   True**   This is a typical feature. The ESR and levels of muscle enzymes are raised in proportion to the degree of active muscle involvement.

**E   False**   There is no absolutely diagnostic test, and diagnosis rests on clinical features supported by investigations. Biopsy of affected sites shows a relatively non-specific perivasculitis.

**G19   A   True**   Basilar artery migraine can cause all manner of brain stem symptoms and signs, including vertigo, nystagmus and even coma.

**B** **True** Friedreich's ataxia is one of the inherited spinocerebellar degenerations. Nystagmus is a common feature due to involvement of spinocerebellar tracts. Corticospinal tracts and posterior columns are also affected.

**C** **True** Most drugs capable of central nervous system depression can cause nystagmus as a toxic effect. Phenytoin is probably one of the commonest to do this in everyday paediatric practice because of its use in epilepsy.

**D** **True** Any severe congenital visual defect such as cataracts or choroidoretinitis can cause optic nystagmus. This differs from cerebellar and vestibular nystagmus in that it is rotary in character, presumably due to inability to fixate.

**E** **False** Guillain–Barré syndrome does not cause nystagmus.

**G20** **A** **False** Although blanket prohibitions of the type were once fashionable in the management of epilepsy, most paediatricians now adopt a policy of common sense precautions aimed at allowing the child to live as normal a life as possible. In the case of swimming, this is usually permitted providing the child is supervised closely by a responsible adult.

**B** **False** Phenytoin causes gum hyperplasia, which is not a recognized side effect of phenobarbitone. The latter drug is famous (perhaps unjustly) for causing hyperactivity and behaviour disorders in young children. A recent study has shown that the difference between phenobarbitone and placebo in this respect was much less than expected, suggesting that much of the behavioural disturbance seen in the past was probably a result of the emotional trauma associated with hospitalization.

**C** **True** Infantile (salaam) spasms (West syndrome) are a clinical syndrome not a specific diagnosis. They are a manifestation of epilepsy, occur mainly during the first 2 years of life and are often associated with a poor prognosis for normal development. Tuberous sclerosis often presents with infantile spasms. ACTH or prednisolone were the drugs of first choice in this condition for many years, but may be about to be superseded by vigabatrin.

**D    False**    Most children with epilepsy should be educated in normal schools, and it is the responsibility of the doctor to facilitate this by educating and reassuring teaching staff concerning the management of possible future convulsions.

**E    False**    Most authorities accept that anticonvulsant medication should only be offered after a *second* convulsion, not a first. Part of the rationale for this is the possibility that the first convulsion was a response to a non-recurrent illness, e.g. a subclinical viral meningoencephalitis. Certainly most doctors would offer anticonvulsant medication after a second convulsion and for a duration of 2–3 years, but even then it is not necessarily a major tragedy if parents respectfully decline this offer.

# PAPER H
## QUESTIONS

**H1** In examination of the cardiovascular system:
  A   an apex beat displaced to the left is pathognomonic of left ventricular hypertrophy.
  B   a pansystolic murmur at the left sternal edge may be associated with a pulsatile liver.
  C   splitting of the second sound is widened in pulmonary hypertension.
  D   the murmur of pulmonary incompetence is very similar to the murmur of mitral incompetence.
  E   the characteristic murmur of aortic stenosis is a pansystolic murmur in the aortic area.

**H2** Concerning fluid and electrolyte balance in children:
  A   daily maintenance requirements for sodium are greater than for potassium.
  B   the incidence of hypertonic dehydration in the UK is decreasing.
  C   an infant with hypertonic dehydration is less likely to show the features of clinical dehydration than an infant with isotonic dehydration with the same fluid deficit.
  D   the emergency treatment of hypertonic dehydration includes rapid infusion of 20 ml/kg, 4% dextrose in 0.18% saline.
  E   all children with more than 5% dehydration need intravenous fluids.

**H3** Anhidrotic ectodermal dysplasia has the following features:
  A   autosomal recessive inheritance.
  B   liability to heat stroke.
  C   scanty hair and eyebrows.
  D   hypercalcaemia.
  E   cyclical neutropenia.

**H4** Cystic fibrosis:
  A   can be diagnosed prenatally by amniocentesis.
  B   characteristically presents in the neonatal period with necrotizing enterocolitis.
  C   is characteristically associated with congenital heart disease.

D   has a recognized association with polycystic kidneys.
E   can cause biliary cirrhosis.

**H5   In the Stevens–Johnson syndrome (severe bullous erythema multiforme):**
A   there is a recognized association with *Mycoplasma pneumoniae* infection.
B   target lesions are characteristic.
C   eye involvement may lead to blindness.
D   steroids are contraindicated.
E   sudden death from myocardial infarction may occur in the convalescent period.

**H6   Prolonged neonatal jaundice is a recognized feature in infants with:**
A   cytomegalovirus (CMV) infection.
B   congenital hypothyroidism.
C   an untreated urinary tract infection.
D   tracheo-oesophageal fistula.
E   galactosaemia.

**H7   In a child with primary pulmonary tuberculosis (TB):**
A   diagnosis depends on finding acid-fast bacilli (AFB) in sputum.
B   the Mantoux test is likely to be strongly positive.
C   the child should be kept off school for the first 6 weeks of treatment.
D   the most likely source of infection is another child.
E   haemoptysis is the most likely prominent symptom.

**H8   Henoch–Schönlein syndrome:**
A   is rare under the age of 1 year.
B   may cause intussusception.
C   has a rash which is characteristically over the flexor surfaces of the limbs.
D   causes thrombocytopenia.
E   responds well to steroid therapy as regards abdominal symptoms.

**H9   An upper motor neuron lesion hemiparesis:**
A   results in flexion of the wrist and elbow.
B   may be associated with wasting.
C   involves the anterior horn cell.
D   may be a cause of foot drop.
E   produces fasciculation.

**H10   The following infectious diseases are associated with a recognized complication:**
A   varicella: myocarditis.
B   rubella: thrombocytopenia.
C   scarlet fever: protein-losing enteropathy.

**D** measles: encephalitis.
**E** meningococcal septicaemia: disseminated intravascular coagulation.

**H11** **In a baby of 32 weeks' gestation who has tachypnoea and sternal recession at 4 hours of age:**
**A** the ductus arteriosus is likely to be patent.
**B** meconium aspiration pneumonia is a likely diagnosis.
**C** the L:S (lecithin: sphingomyelin) ratio is likely to be low.
**D** fluid levels on the chest X-ray suggest pneumonia due to group B *Streptococcus*.
**E** the presence of bowel shadows on the left side of the chest on X-ray is diagnostic of tracheo-oesophageal fistula.

**H12** **In the detection and management of congenital dislocation of the hip (CDH):**
**A** all 'clicky' hips should be followed up till the age of 2 years.
**B** abduction splinting can result in avascular necrosis of the femoral head.
**C** the optimum time for screening is the first birthday check.
**D** abduction to 180° excludes a dislocatable hip.
**E** there is a higher incidence of the condition in Africa.

**H13** **In ventricular septal defect (VSD):**
**A** the smallest defects tend to produce the softest murmurs.
**B** left-to-right shunting leads to increased risk of cerebral abscess.
**C** there may be a diastolic murmur at the apex.
**D** the systolic murmur increases in intensity as pulmonary hypertension develops.
**E** there is no risk of bacterial endocarditis.

**H14** **Recurrent aphthous ulcers in children are a recognized association of:**
**A** eczema.
**B** Crohn's disease.
**C** sickle cell anaemia.
**D** coeliac disease.
**E** the use of fluoride toothpaste.

**H15** **Pancreatic insufficiency:**
**A** has a recognized association with cyclical neutropenia.
**B** has a recognized association with bronchiectasis.
**C** characteristically reduces absorption of medium chain triglycerides (MCTs).
**D** causes subtotal villous atrophy.
**E** is likely to give an impaired xylose absorption test.

**H16** **In hypoparathyroidism:**
A  constipation is a characteristic feature.
B  parathormone is the treatment of choice.
C  there may be intracranial calcification.
D  there may be an associated immune deficiency state.
E  there may be an increased incidence of fungal skin infections.

**H17** **In congenital adrenal hyperplasia:**
A  a male infant may appear normal at birth.
B  testicular hypertrophy occurs.
C  a female infant typically has clitoral hypertrophy and fusion of the labia minora.
D  infants may present with shock in the early weeks of life.
E  ACTH is an effective treatment.

**H18** **Febrile convulsions:**
A  characteristically occur on the second day of a feverish episode.
B  can usefully be treated by sodium valproate per rectum.
C  can usefully be treated by intramuscular diazepam.
D  are best prevented by long-term phenytoin therapy.
E  have a peak incidence between the ages of 3 months and 1 year.

**H19** **Disseminated intravascular coagulation (DIC):**
A  is excluded as a diagnosis by the absence of fibrin degradation products (FDPs).
B  responds to early treatment with vitamin K.
C  may be caused by hyperpyrexia.
D  may benefit from treatment with fresh frozen plasma.
E  may occur in malaria due to *Plasmodium falciparum*.

**H20** **The following are true of pseudohypertrophic (Duchenne) muscular dystrophy:**
A  there is an increased incidence of mild mental handicap in children with the condition.
B  the condition is usually symptom-free under the age of 5 years.
C  normal serum creatine kinase in a female relative excludes the carrier state.
D  pseudohypertrophy correlates with improved prognosis.
E  mutations are responsible for about 30% of new cases.

# PAPER H
## ANSWERS

**H1** **A** **False** Displacement of the apex beat is *not* pathognomonic of left ventricular hypertrophy (LVH). It may signify *dilatation* of the left ventricle without muscular hypertrophy (as in cardiomyopathy). It may simply signify mediastinal shift (as in left lower lobe collapse, large right side pleural effusion, etc.). The cardinal sign of LVH is a *thrusting* apex and this remains true even if the apex is not displaced, e.g. in aortic stenosis.

    **B** **True** Such a murmur is characteristic of tricuspid incompetence which is a cause of a pulsatile liver. In addition, one should expect to see prominent 'v' waves in the neck. Tricuspid incompetence is a feature of Ebstein's anomaly and can also occur in conditions causing dilatation of the right ventricle, e.g. severe pulmonary hypertension, cardiomyopathy.

    **C** **False** The two main signs of pulmonary hypertension are (1) loud pulmonary component of the second sound and (2) right ventricular hypertrophy. With regard to changes in splitting of the second sound, the split will be narrower not wider, because the pressure difference between the systemic and pulmonary aorta will be reduced.

    **D** **False** Pulmonary incompetence gives a high-pitched soft early diastolic murmur at the lower left sternal edge which is virtually identical to that of aortic incompetence. Mitral incompetence gives a blowing pansystolic murmur at the apex radiating to the axilla.

    **E** **False** Only three conditions give pansystolic murmurs: mitral incompetence, tricuspid incompetence and ventricular septal defect. The murmur of aortic stenosis is a rough *ejection* systolic murmur which is maximal in the aortic area but radiates to both the apex and the right side of the neck.

**H2    A    False**    Surprisingly, despite the great difference in their serum levels, the daily maintenance requirements for sodium and potassium are approximately identical at 2–3 meq/kg/24 hours, throughout childhood. This reflects the kidney's far greater ability to conserve sodium compared with potassium.

**B    True**    There was great concern about the rising incidence of hypertonic dehydration in the late 1960s. The incidence began to fall in the early 1970s and has continued to do so, probably due to a major campaign of health education aimed at telling mothers not to heap up or add extra scoops of powdered milk, and to give extra water during febrile episodes.

**C    True**    In hypertonic dehydration the main deficit is water not sodium, and this deficiency of water is spread through all the body compartments including the largest, viz. the intracellular compartment. The extracellular fluid (ECF) volume is therefore nearly normal until very late in the disease. As the signs of 'clinical dehydration' are mainly those of ECF volume depletion the child with hypertonic dehydration does not usually look dehydrated. In contrast, isotonic dehydration is virtually synonymous with ECF depletion which is directly reflected in decreased tissue turgor, sunken eyes and decreased venous filling.

**D    False**    4% dextrose in 0.18% saline contains 31 mmol/litre of $Na^+$. To infuse any quantity of this rapidly into a normal person would be dangerous but even more so if the patient already had hypertonic dehydration. There would be a risk of a rapid drop in serum $Na^+$ and a rapid increase in intracellular water, with the danger of convulsions and cerebral oedema. The formula '20 ml/kg fast' was devised for blood or plasma in haemorrhagic or hypovolaemic shock as it constitutes roughly 25% of the blood volume. If 0.9% saline is used in severe isotonic dehydration, 20 ml/kg will not be enough for resuscitation as most of it will leave the vascular compartment and equilibrate with the interstitial fluid.

**E** **False** Oral rehydration has been shown to be remarkably effective in preventing and treating severe dehydration in all forms of gastroenteritis and cholera. It can be used as the initial treatment in most children with 5–10% dehydration. It depends on the ability of glucose and sodium to be actively transported together across the small intestinal mucosa, together with water. Appropriate solutions contain sucrose or glucose plus 70–90 mmol/litre $Na^+$ together with added potassium and bicarbonate. Many proprietary preparations only contain sodium concentrations of 40–60 mmol/l and are therefore not appropriate for true rehydration therapy.

**H3** **A** **False** Anhidrotic ectodermal dysplasia is probably inherited as a sex-linked recessive, the majority of cases occurring in males.

**B** **True** Liability to heat stroke is the most important clinical implication of a diagnosis of anhidrotic ectodermal dysplasia. In this condition there is incomplete development of the epidermis and its appendages including sweat glands. Subjects are virtually unable to sweat, rendering them liable to heat stroke during febrile illnesses and heat waves. They may present with prolonged febrile convulsions.

**C** **True** In this condition the hair is sparse and easily pulled out. The eyebrows are scanty, there are prominent supraorbital ridges and ears, and thick protruding lips, all of which gives these children a characteristic appearance.

**D** **False** Hypercalcaemia is not a recognized feature of this condition. Although the teeth are poorly formed and liable to caries, this is not due to any defect in calcium metabolism.

**E** **False** Cyclical neutropenia is not a recognized association of anhidrotic ectodermal dysplasia. It can occur on its own as an isolated phenomenon, or else in association with pancreatic insufficiency (the Schwackman–Diamond syndrome).

**H4** **A** **False** Amniocentesis has nothing to offer in this area. Chorionic villous blood sampling *can* give diagnostic information if the particular gene in the family has been identified.

**B   False**   The common gut presentation of cystic fibrosis is with meconium ileus. Necrotizing enterocolitis is a different disease entity of unknown aetiology, occurring in preterm infants and carrying a high mortality and morbidity.

**C   False**   There is no association between cystic fibrosis and congenital heart disease.

**D   False**   Polycystic kidneys have an association with congenital hepatic fibrosis. Cystic fibrosis causes biliary cirrhosis. However these liver conditions are different disease entities and there is no association between cystic fibrosis and polycystic kidneys.

**E   True**   Cystic fibrosis causes biliary cirrhosis because of obstruction of the biliary tree by the tenacious secretions common in this condition.

**H5   A   True**   *Mycoplasma pneumoniae* infection is one of the commonest positive associations with this condition in clinical practice.

**B   True**   The target lesion consists of an erythematous ring with a paler inner ring with a central vesicle.

**C   True**   A severe conjunctivitis with secondary bacterial infection may lead to corneal damage and blindness. Significant eye involvement is a definite indication for systemic steroid therapy.

**D   False**   See (C).

**E   False**   This statement is true for the mucocutaneous lymph node syndrome (MCLS, Kawasaki disease) which resembles the Stevens–Johnson syndrome in some of its clinical features.

**H6   A   True**   Congenital CMV infection is a recognized cause of neonatal hepatitis.

**B   True**   Congenital hypothyroidism is associated with a prolonged unconjugated hyperbilirubinaemia.

**C   True**   Any low-grade continuing bacterial or viral infection can cause prolongation of neonatal jaundice.

**D   False**

**E   True**   Like hypothyroidism, galactosaemia is a preventable cause of severe mental retardation which it is vital not to miss in the neonatal period. Urine should be tested for reducing substances with Clinitest.

**H7**  **A**  **False**  Primary TB differs radically from post-primary TB in several ways, the most striking being the fact that in the former bacilli are scanty and in the latter numerous. In primary pulmonary TB the inhaled organisms lead to the primary focus and then spread to the local lymph nodes where the infection usually stops. The child may have malaise, fever and weight loss but cough and sputum are usually insignificant. The diagnosis is usually made on the clinical picture, chest X-ray and positive Mantoux test. Enthusiasm for recovering AFB from gastric washings is misplaced and should not delay diagnosis and treatment.

  **B**  **True**

  **C**  **False**  Uncomplicated primary TB is not infectious. Even if it had progressed to the post-primary stage, and infective sputum was being produced, appropriate drug therapy would render the child non-infective within a week. Treatment is given because of the small risk (c. 2%) of progress of the infection.

  **D**  **False**  Adults with post-primary pulmonary TB are by far the most likely source of infections, and are usually relatives.

  **E**  **False**  Haemoptysis is a feature of post-primary pulmonary TB, see (A).

**H8**  **A**  **True**  The disease is most common among pre-school children but is rare in the first year of life.

  **B**  **True**  Intussusception is a relatively rare complication of the syndrome. More commonly there is simple haemorrhage into the gut wall with colicky abdominal pain, vomiting and melaena.

  **C**  **False**  The rash, which is either urticarial or purpuric, is characteristically over extensor surfaces, especially the buttocks, backs of the thighs and dorsum of the feet.

  **D**  **False**  Purpura in this condition is due to a vasculitis, and thrombocytopenia is not a feature.

  **E**  **True**  Renal involvement, whether acute nephritis, nephrotic syndrome or chronic renal failure, shows no response whatsoever to steroid therapy. However, abdominal symptoms usually respond well to steroids, which are perfectly justifiable therapy if the child is suffering.

**H9**   **A**   **True**   When a limb is rendered spastic, the stronger muscle groups predominate. Thus a child with hemiplegic cerebral palsy has an arm fixed in flexion (of the wrist and elbow). In the leg, hip and knee extension and foot plantar flexion predominate.

**B**   **False**   In upper motor neuron lesions the muscles remain innervated and hypertonic therefore there is no wasting. Wasting only occurs in lower motor neuron lesions, muscle disease or disuse.

**C**   **False**

**D**   **True**   See (A).

**E**   **False**   Fasciculation is a sign of ongoing anterior horn cell degeneration (as in spinal muscular atrophy).

**H10**   **A**   **True**   Varicella usually causes only a mild illness in childhood with few complications, the commonest being an encephalitis which mainly affects the cerebellum. In susceptible adults it tends to cause a more severe illness which may include myocarditis as one of the complications. A diffuse pneumonia may also occur which may leave fine specks of calcification on subsequent X-rays.

**B**   **True**   Rubella is usually a very mild illness, and the rash usually appears on the first day of the illness. Enlargement of posterior auricular and occipital lymph nodes is common. Complications are rare but they include thrombocytopenia and encephalitis.

**C**   **False**   Scarlet fever consists of a streptococcal infection, usually tonsillitis, with an associated erythematous rash due to streptococcal exotoxin. Clinically and epidemiologically it is of no greater importance than an attack of tonsillitis without the rash. Rheumatic fever and acute nephritis are rare complications. Protein-losing enteropathy is not a recognized complication.

**D**   **True**   Encephalitis is a relatively common and potentially serious complication of measles, and constitutes one of the main justifications for immunization of the childhood population against measles. Encephalitis is said to occur in 1 in 1000 cases of measles, and to carry a mortality of 15%, with 25% of cases suffering a degree of brain damage. This acute encephalitis is distinct from the much later and extremely rare condition of subacute sclerosing panencephalitis which is, however, also thought to be a late consequence of measles infection.

**E** **True** Virtually any infectious disease is capable of causing disseminated intravascular coagulation (DIC). Meningococcal septicaemia is one of the diseases most likely to do so. This complication is much to be feared, as it can cause fulminating deterioration and death even in cases receiving early medical attention. It should be suspected if there is a petechial or purpuric rash, unexpected bleeding from puncture sites or peripheral circulatory failure. Blood tests will reveal thrombocytopenia and anaemia with characteristically crenated red cells on blood film. In addition there may be a generalized disorder of coagulation due to consumption of clotting factors, with a low serum fibrinogen and raised fibrin degradation products (FDPs). Treatment is by replacement of plasma volume (with plasma), blood transfusion and fresh frozen plasma and platelets if necessary.

**H11** **A** **True** The duct is quite likely to be patent in any 32-week infant aged 4 hours. The additional presence of respiratory distress makes its continued patency even more likely as there may be hypoxaemia and increased pulmonary vascular resistance.

**B** **False** Meconium aspiration is a disease of asphyxiated term infants, and is virtually unknown in infants of 32 weeks' gestation.

**C** **True** The most likely diagnosis is hyaline membrane disease, in which low L:S ratios are characteristic.

**D** **False** The chest X-ray in Group B streptococcal pneumonia is characteristically of ground glass or patchy opacities bilaterally. Fluid levels are seen as a result of infection with *Staphylococcus aureus*, which classically causes scattered microabscesses. These would be unlikely to develop by 4 hours.

**E** **False** These X-ray findings suggest diaphragmatic hernia and there is likely to be acquired dextrocardia. The chest X-ray in tracheo-oesophageal fistula may look normal and the diagnosis depends on failure to pass a wide-bored tube into the stomach.

**H12** **A** **False** A lot of 'clicks' are innocent and ligamentous in origin, and a competent examiner can exclude either a dislocated or a dislocatable hip outright. To follow up all these cases is a waste of time for doctors and mothers alike.

**B  True**    This is one of the unfortunate side effects of treatment, and has led to a loss of popularity for extreme degrees of abduction in treatment. It is also possible that over-enthusiastic attempts to manipulate a dislocated hip can cause this complication.

**C  False**   A hip that remains dislocated for the first year of life is a tragedy, as it will never be entirely normal. Manipulation with or without corrective surgery may achieve reduction, but the abnormal architecture will predispose to almost certain premature osteoarthritis. CDH should be detected in the first week of life and treated immediately. It is desirable that clinic doctors repeatedly check the hips at each attendance in the first 6 months of life to pick up the small number of cases that are missed at the neonatal check.

**D  False**   If the hips can be abducted to 180° they are not *dislocated* at that moment in time. However, they may have been dislocated at the onset of the manoeuvre and 'clunked' back into position during abduction. Even if the hips are not dislocated, abduction to 180° will not exclude their being *dislocatable*, which must be tested for separately by attempting (gently) to dislocate the hip by backward pressure to the flexed hip.

**E  False**   CDH is very rare in Africa. This is probably due to a combination of genetic factors and the therapeutic value of mothers carrying their infants strapped to their backs with hips flexed and abducted.

**H13  A  False**   The loudness of the murmur in VSD is proportional to the velocity of the jet of blood flowing across the defect. Thus small defects ('maladie de Roger') produce the loudest murmurs and are the more likely to produce a thrill.

**B  False**   Left-to-right shunts carry no increased risk of cerebral abscess whereas right-to-left shunts do, because the filtering effect of the lungs on bacteria in systemic venous blood is bypassed.

**C  True**    When left-to-right shunting is significant in VSD there is increased flow across the mitral valve and this may result in a mid-diastolic flow murmur at the apex.

**D  False**   As pulmonary hypertension develops the pressure gradient between left and right is reduced, and the systolic murmur reduces in intensity and may become shorter.

E **False** There is a significant risk of endocarditis in even the smallest ventricular septal defects. Atrial septal defect is said to carry virtually no risk of endocarditis.

**H14** A **False** Recurrent aphthous stomatitis can be a distressing and troublesome disorder in which often no underlying diagnosis is found. There is no recognized association with eczema.

B **True** Aphthous stomatitis is a recognized association of Crohn's disease, and also of ulcerative colitis.

C **False**

D **True** Coeliac disease and recurrent aphthous ulceration are recognized associations. Gluten-free diet leads to cure of both conditions. Some cases of recurrent aphthous ulceration *not* associated with coeliac disease do respond to dietary exclusion regimes, both of gluten and other foods.

E **False**

**H15** A **True** The so-called Schwackman–Diamond syndrome. These children present with failure to thrive in early infancy. Management consists of pancreatic supplements, with the possible addition of prophylactic antibiotics during periods of neutropenia.

B **True** In cystic fibrosis.

C **False** MCTs are absorbed directly by the small intestine without prior digestion, and are in fact used for this purpose in aiding nutrition in patients with pancreatic insufficiency.

D **False**

E **False** Xylose absorption is impaired in diseases affecting the small bowel mucosa, e.g. coeliac disease, Crohn's disease. Pancreatic insufficiency with a normal small bowel will therefore not affect xylose absorption.

**H16** A **False** Hypoparathyroidism causes hypocalcaemia which tends to cause diarrhoea. Hypercalcaemia causes constipation.

B **False** While parathormone is effective in raising the serum calcium in hypoparathyroidism it needs to be given intravenously. The treatment of choice is high-dose oral vitamin D, which increases calcium absorption from the gut.

**C  True**   The calcification is characteristically in the basal ganglia. Hypocalcaemia needs to be prolonged and untreated to result in these changes, and usually there will be associated cataracts and mental retardation.

**D  True**   In the branchial arch defect syndrome (DiGeorge syndrome) there is a combination of immune deficiency (due to lymphopenia and thymic aplasia) with hypoparathyroidism with the additional possibility of congenital heart disease. This combination of defects is thought to be due to the fact that all the defective structures arise from the third and fourth branchial arches.

**E  True**   This association is a recognized part of the DiGeorge syndrome and is a reflection of the decreased cellular immunity. It does not occur in idiopathic simple hypoparathyroidism.

**H17  A  True**   Congenital adrenal hyperplasia consists of a group of related conditions inherited as autosomal recessives. Their basic feature is a missing enzyme necessary for one of the steps in the synthesis of cortisol and aldosterone. The deficiency of these hormones leads to raised endogenous ACTH which results in increased androgen secretion by the adrenal cortex. This produces masculinization of female infants, but male infants may appear normal at birth which unfortunately leads to delays in diagnosis.

**B  False**   Excess androgens cause increased secondary sexual characteristics only. Testicular hypertrophy can occur only in response to pituitary gonadotrophins which are not elevated in this condition.

**C  True**   The actions of androgens in the antenatal period produce an already virilized female infant with clitoral hypertrophy and fusion of the labia minora. If this process is extreme the infant may be mistaken for a male infant with cryptorchidism and hypospadias.

**D  True**   These infants essentially have adrenocortical insufficiency. They accordingly fail to thrive, and if serum electrolytes are estimated these reveal a low sodium and high potassium. Unless diagnosed and treated these infants may sink into an Addisonian crisis with shock as the main feature, which requires urgent treatment consisting of intravenous 0.9% saline, hydrocortisone and added glucose.

E   **False**   These infants already have high endogenous ACTH levels which are unable to generate synthesis of endogenous glucocorticoids and mineralocorticoids. ACTH is therefore totally ineffective therapy. Instead, infants should receive maintenance hydrocortisone and fludrocortisone for life. Any illness episode should be covered by increased hydrocortisone in the normal way.

H18   A   **False**   Febrile convulsions characteristically occur during the *initial* period of the onset of a fever, and are surprisingly uncommon on subsequent days. This feature makes them difficult to anticipate and sometimes means that the presence of significant pyrexia is appreciated only after the convulsion has occurred.

B   **False**   While some studies have shown that sodium valproate is an effective prophylactic drug, it is not an appropriate drug for emergency treatment by this or any other route.

C   **False**   Diazepam given intramuscularly is poorly and erratically absorbed into the circulation and is not to be recommended. Intravenous diazepam has long been the emergency treatment of choice for febrile and non-febrile convulsions. It has also been shown that the rectal route is very effective, giving therapeutic blood levels in 10–15 minutes. This refers to diazepam being administered in a fluid form, not as a suppository. The practical problems of finding a vein in convulsing toddlers increase the attractions of this alternative. Increasingly, parents are being given rectal diazepam for emergency use outside hospital.

D   **False**   While there have been numerous and conflicting trials on different drugs for the prophylaxis of febrile convulsions, there is reasonable agreement that phenytoin is *not* the drug of choice in this area, on the grounds of general lack of efficacy. Phenobarbitone or sodium valporate are probably the drugs of first choice if continuous therapy is decided upon.

E   **False**   The incidence of febrile convulsions starts from virtually zero at 6 months to a peak at 18–24 months of age, reflecting the parallel between increasing differentiation of the brain and its susceptibility to insult. Below 6 months of age the brain is very resistant to insult and convulsions occurring at this age should be viewed with suspicion as they may reflect organic pathology.

**H19** **A** **False** DIC can be either a self-limiting condition or a rapidly progressive condition with a high mortality. Early diagnosis can be made on the characteristic appearances of the blood film (fragmented or 'burr' cells) together with evidence of a falling platelet count. Fibrin degradation products may be absent in the early stages of the condition.

**B** **False** Theoretically treatment with heparin might be beneficial in the early stages of the condition, but evidence as to its usefulness in clinical practice is difficult to find.

**C** **True** Severe hyperpyrexia in infants can cause convulsions, shock, brain damage, disseminated intravascular coagulation and death, and has been implicated as a cause of cot deaths.

**D** **True** In the established case of DIC there is consumption of all clotting factors, and replacement therapy with fresh frozen plasma is indicated. Fresh whole blood and platelet transfusion may also be indicated.

**E** **True** DIC has been described in a wide variety of bacterial, viral and protozoal diseases, including falciparum malaria. Meningococcal septicaemia is the bacterial infection most likely to cause this condition.

**H20** **A** **True**

**B** **False** It should be perfectly possible to diagnose affected children from about the age of 2–3 years onwards. Failure to diagnose cases until they are over the age of 5 years is regrettably common and often denies the family early genetic counselling. Late walking is characteristic, as is an unsteady gait and difficulty in climbing stairs.

**C** **False** A raised creatine kinase (CK) means the mother is a carrier. However, a normal CK does not exclude the carrier state and DNA analysis is needed for a definite answer.

**D** **False** Pseudohypertrophy is of no prognostic significance.

**E** **True**

# PAPER I
## QUESTIONS

**I1**  **Regarding lung development:**
  A   the maximum number of alveoli are present by the time of birth.
  B   the pulmonary hypoplasia in Potter syndrome is secondary to lung compression due to oligohydramnios.
  C   congenital diaphragmatic hernia is commonly associated with a degree of pulmonary hypoplasia.
  D   adenovirus infection can result in bronchiolitis obliterans.
  E   significant alveolar development is present by 20 weeks' gestation.

**I2**  **Regarding chromosomal disorders:**
  A   a de novo balanced reciprocal translocation identified on routine amniocentesis conveys a 50% risk of mental handicap.
  B   some male carriers of Robertsonian t(13:14) translocations present with infertility due to a low sperm count.
  C   trisomy 21 accounts for approximately 95% of Down syndrome cases.
  D   blood chromosomal analysis should be performed on any dysmorphic baby even if an amniocentesis on the baby showed normal chromosomes.
  E   parents of children with Wolf–Hirschorn syndrome (4p-) should have their chromosomes checked.

**I3**  **The following are recognized associations:**
  A   lymphoid interstitial pneumonia and HIV infection.
  B   specific antibody deficiency and recurrent otitis media.
  C   haemoptysis and cystic fibrosis.
  D   bronchiectasis and chronic sinusitis.
  E   blood-stained pericardial fluid and tuberculosis.

**I4**  **A parietal lobe lesion is characteristically associated with:**
  A   disinhibition.
  B   dysphasia.
  C   dressing apraxia.
  D   sensory inattention.
  E   superior quadrantanopia visual field defect.

**I5** **The following is true of Lyme disease:**
- A  the causative organism is a rickettsia.
- B  the name comes from Lyme Regis in Dorset.
- C  the classical rash of this condition occurs 2–3 months after initial infection.
- D  neurological features are dramatically reversed by antibiotic treatment.
- E  inflammation of mucocutaneous junctions is a cardinal feature.

**I6** **Regarding blood gas results, the following statements are true:**
- A  levels of $PCO_2$ below 3.3 kPa can be harmful.
- B  carbon dioxide is twice as diffusible as oxygen.
- C  in an ill child with advanced lung damage due to cystic fibrosis and a pH of 7.38, $PCO_2$ 9.1 kPa and a $PO_2$ of 3.5 kPa, it would be appropriate to give 80% oxygen via face mask.
- D  $PCO_2$ values need to be corrected if capillary sampling is used.
- E  in a breathless child with asthma a $pco_2$ level of 3 kPa with a $PO_2$ of 7 kPa is likely to be due to generalized alveolar hypoventilation.

**I7** **Asperger syndrome:**
- A  should not be diagnosed if speech and language development is delayed.
- B  is commonly associated with gross and fine motor incoordination.
- C  is associated with an acute over-sensitivity to the feelings of others.
- D  is easy to misdiagnose as due to abnormal parenting.
- E  typically shows improvement with age through childhood and adolescence.

**I8** **The following are true of Munchausen syndrome by proxy:**
- A  fathers are as likely to be responsible as mothers.
- B  the symptoms only occur in the presence of the parent.
- C  the parent responsible will often have had connections with the medical profession.
- D  the commonest pattern is that the child is presented with a complaint of symptoms which are different on each occasion.
- E  the prognosis is essentially benign in the majority of cases.

**I9** ***Pneumocystis carinii* infection in children:**
- A  can be treated with nebulized pentamidine.
- B  is commonly acquired from contaminated water supplies.
- C  radiological changes are often more severe than the clinical changes would suggest.

**D** only occurs in children who have received immunosuppressive drugs.
**E** co-amoxiclav (Augmentin) is the prophylactic drug of choice.

**I10** **Patent ductus arteriosus (PDA) in the preterm infant:**
**A** presents clinically earlier in infants treated with surfactant.
**B** is a recognized risk factor for pulmonary haemorrhage.
**C** responds to indomethacin in over 90% of cases.
**D** if untreated can increase the risk of bronchopulmonary dysplasia (BDP).
**E** in infants under 1000 g, indomethacin treatment should be reserved for those who are symptomatic.

**I11** **The following are characteristic features of innocent murmurs in childhood:**
**A** occurrence in diastole.
**B** quiet (i.e. soft) murmurs.
**C** maximally heard at apex.
**D** a venous hum is best heard at the lower left sternal edge.
**E** more likely to be heard if child is feverish.

**I12** **Sudden withdrawal of long-term oral steroid therapy in children can cause:**
**A** hypernatraemia.
**B** hyperkalaemia.
**C** petechial haemorrhage.
**D** postural hypotension.
**E** diabetes mellitus.

**I13** **A lesion of the right VIth cranial nerve:**
**A** can cause diplopia when looking to the left.
**B** can cause a convergent strabismus.
**C** neither eye will be able to cross the midline.
**D** causes diplopia with the images separating further on gaze to the right.
**E** may be due to raised intracranial pressure.

**I14** **Recognized presenting features of severe combined immunodeficiency (SCID) include:**
**A** persistent cutaneous candidiasis.
**B** *Pneumocystis carinii* pneumonia.
**C** granuloma formation.
**D** a family history of unexplained deaths in siblings.
**E** reversed CD4:CD8 ratio.

**I15** **In assessing the development of a child aged 3 years, one would expect him/her to be able to:**
**A** talk in sentences.
**B** recognize three colours.

C tolerate admission to hospital for 48 hours without parents being resident.
D write his/her name.
E enjoy make-believe play.

**I16 Cleft lip and palate are associated with:**
A hearing difficulties.
B maternal anticonvulsant therapy.
C pseudohypoparathyroidism.
D cardiac defects.
E micrognathia.

**I17 Idiopathic thrombocytopenic purpura (ITP):**
A carries a 1% risk of intracranial haemorrhage if the platelet count falls below $20 \times 10^9$/l.
B should be treated by splenectomy if the platelet count is less than $10 \times 10^9$/l.
C is due to impaired platelet production by the bone marrow.
D bone marrow examination is essential if immunoglobulin treatment is to be used.
E resolves spontaneously within six months in the majority of childhood cases.

**I18 The following conditions characteristically cause jaundice within the first 24 hours of life:**
A glucose 6 phosphate dehydrogenase (G6PD) deficiency.
B congenital hypothyroidism.
C severe congenital cytomegalovirus (CMV) infection.
D choledochal cyst.
E primary tyrosinaemia.

**I19 The following are true of Reye syndrome:**
A jaundice is a common early feature.
B the incidence has declined markedly since the mid 1980s.
C early treatment with acyclovir is beneficial.
D liver biopsy is unlikely to affect management.
E mannitol may be useful in management.

**I20 In a 2-year-old child who had a urinary tract infection, a dimercaptosuccinic acid (DMSA) scan performed within two weeks:**
A can be used to demonstrate the rate of drainage of urine into the bladder.
B will demonstrate the detailed anatomy of the calyces.
C should be a second line imaging investigation because of its high radiation dose.
D any areas of focal scarring caused by a UTI (reflux nephropathy) are likely to be visible.
E may demonstrate areas of focal inflammation that can fully resolve.

# PAPER I
## ANSWERS

**I1**  **A**  **False**  The number of alveoli increases approximately 10-fold in the first 8 years of life.

**B**  **False**  The pulmonary hypoplasia occurs earlier in pregnancy than can be explained as due to a mechanical effect from oligohydramnios. It is thought that the kidney normally produces a factor to promote lung growth and that this is lacking in Potter syndrome.

**C**  **True**  The mechanism here *is* thought to be mainly mechanical.

**D**  **True**  Bronchiolitis obliterans is a rare complication of adenovirus pneumonia in the first few years of life. It may be misdiagnosed as severe asthma relatively resistant to treatment.

**E**  **False**  Up to 20 weeks' gestation the airways are just beginning to canalize, and there is no significant alveolar development until 20–24 weeks.

**I2**  **A**  **False**  The risk is 10%.

**B**  **True**

**C**  **True**

**D**  **True**  Blood chromosomal analysis gives a superior quality preparation; subtle chromosomal abnormalities may require blood chromosomal preparations in order to be identified.

**E**  **True**  In 5% of cases one or other parent may be carrying a balanced reciprocal translocation which has resulted in the deletion.

**I3**  **A**  **True**

**B**  **True**  In particular, subgroup IgG deficiencies can often be demonstrated in this group of children. Prophylaxis with cotrimoxazole for 6–12-month periods has been shown to be very effective.

C   **True**

D   **True**   Via the mechanism of primary ciliary dyskinesia. 50% of these cases have dextrocardia, in which case they constitute Kartagener syndrome.

E   **True**

I4   A   **False**   Disinhibition (i.e. socially inappropriate behaviour) in association with personality change is typical of frontal lobe pathology.

B   **True**   Dysphasia results from lesions of the dominant (usually left) parietal lobe.

C   **True**   Lesions of the non-dominant parietal lobe can lead to very handicapping problems of visuospatial organization, including dressing apraxia, sensory inattention and astereognosis.

D   **True**   See above.

E   **False**   In practice field defects are very rare with parietal lesions; in theory they would give an inferior quadrantic field defect. A superior quadrantanopia results from temporal lobe lesions.

I5   A   **False**   The causative organism is a spirochaete, *Borrelia burgdorferi*. It is transmitted by the bites of ticks which live on deer (or moose) in the USA and Northern Europe.

B   **False**   The name comes from Lyme in Connecticut where the condition was first recognized in 1975.

C   **False**   The rash (erythema chronicum migrans) occurs in the first stage of the disease, 1–4 weeks after infection. The rash is the vital clue to early diagnosis and treatment.

D   **False**   This condition is best thought of as parallel to syphilis in that in both diseases there can be irreversible damage to the central nervous system in the later stages. In Lyme disease there can be a meningoencephalitis with cranial and peripheral nerve lesions. Myocarditis and an erosive arthropathy can also occur. *Early* diagnosis and antibiotic treatment can protect from all these complications.

E   **False**   This is a feature of Kawasaki disease.

I6   A   **True**   Levels of $P\text{co}_2$ as low as this can lead to cerebral vasoconstriction and hypoperfusion.

B   **False**   $\text{co}_2$ is *ten* times as diffusible as oxygen.

**C** **False** This could be dangerous as the situation is analogous to the adult with cor pulmonale. The respiratory centre has become insensitive to $CO_2$ and respiratory drive is in response to hypoxia. Abolishing hypoxia with generous oxygen therapy could lead to apnoea.

**D** **False** Provided the skin perfusion is good, capillary sampling gives $PCO_2$ levels that correlate well with arterial samples.

**E** **False** This child is maintaining its $PO_2$ by compensatory *hyper*ventilation which is blowing off the more diffusible $CO_2$ (see B). Generalized alveolar hypoventilation causes a raised $PCO_2$.

**I7** **A** **True** Asperger syndrome, while regarded as one of the autistic spectrum disorders, differs from true autism in having near-normal speech and language development. Diagnosis is often delayed in the early years as the child is just regarded as 'quirky', or 'part of nature's rich pattern'.

**B** **True**

**C** **False** Children with this syndrome seem to be oblivious to other people's feelings and needs.

**D** **True** Misdiagnosis along these lines has led to several cases where care proceedings were initiated against parents.

**E** **False** The handicaps these children suffer from become progressively unmasked throughout childhood.

**I8** **A** **False** To date the mother has been the 'guilty' parent in the vast majority of cases.

**B** **True** Characteristically, mothers impress medical and nursing staff by their devotion to their children, spending long periods in hospital with their children while the doctors consider ever more unusual diagnoses. Once the diagnosis is suspected, a trial of parental exclusion will help to confirm it if the symptoms cease to occur.

**C** **True** Nursing and medical receptionist work are among the common associations.

**D** **False** Most commonly, the parent presents the same symptom repeatedly until diagnosis. Common patterns include apnoeic attacks (suffocation), factitious bleeding from various orifices and recurrent unexplained coma or drowsiness (poisoning).

**E   False**   The initial view was that the condition was benign and that it responded to simple confrontation. This is now accepted as over-optimistic, and large series have shown that the prognosis for the child is potentially grave both physically and, especially, psychologically. Munchausen syndrome by proxy should be regarded as a form of child abuse and handled accordingly.

**I9   A   True**   Usually systemic cotrimoxazole would also be used.

**B   False**

**C   True**

**D   False**   *Any* child with compromised immunity is at risk, including children with severe primary immunodeficiencies or HIV infection.

**E   False**   Cotrimoxazole is the prophylactic drug of choice. Co-amoxiclav is not effective.

**I10   A   True**   Surfactant therapy leads to an earlier fall in pulmonary vascular resistance, thus advancing the time at which significant left-to-right shunting occurs.

**B   True**   Pulmonary haemorrhage is the clinical manifestation of haemorrhagic pulmonary oedema, to which PDA predisposes.

**C   False**   The figure is around 70%.

**D   True**

**E   False**   Current orthodoxy is that all infants under 1000 g with PDA should receive a trial of indomethacin.

**I11   A   False**   All diastolic murmurs are significant. Up to 30% of children with normal hearts will have an innocent murmur heard at some stage in childhood. These are either ejection flow murmurs (across normal pulmonary or aortic valves) or venous hums. The former are usually heard best in the pulmonary area or lower left sternal edge, and do not radiate.

**B   True**   A moderately loud pulmonary ejection murmur is more likely to be due to pulmonary stenosis.

**C   False**   See (A).

**D   False**   A venous hum is a continuous low pitched sound best heard below both clavicles. It can be abolished by lying the patient flat or compressing the jugular veins on the same side.

**E** **True** Fever increases cardiac output which will increase turbulence.

**I12** **A** **False** In general, any child (or adult) who is on oral steroids for more than 3 months will suffer decreased function of the pituitary–adrenal axis. Cessation of treatment (or the stress of an infection or operation) can lead to an Addisonian crisis which would be fatal untreated. Features of this will include hyponatraemia, hyperkalaemia, postural hypotension and eventually shock.

**B** **True** See (A).

**C** **False** The association with petechial haemorrhage is in meningococcal septicaemia in which adrenal haemorrhages and possibly Addisonian features may occur terminally. However, an Addisonian state would not *cause* petechial haemorrhages.

**D** **True** See (A).

**E** **False** Oral steroids can *cause* a tendency towards diabetes, but withdrawal would therefore cure it.

**I13** **A** **False** A right VIth (abducens) palsy will paralyse abduction of the right eye, thus its effects will be most marked on looking to the *right*.

**B** **True** Unopposed action of the right medial rectus may result in a convergent strabismus.

**C** **False** The movements of the left eye will be full, and the right eye will have unaffected adduction. The pattern referred to does not occur with simple lesions of the eye muscles, and is instead characteristic of a supranuclear ophthalmoplegia.

**D** **True**

**E** **True** Both IIIrd and VIth nerve palsies can be caused by raised intracranial pressure, the former by compression on the tentorium cerebelli and the latter by stretching. Since the sign is some distance away from the initial lesion, both are examples of a 'false localizing sign'.

**I14** **A** **True** This condition presents in the first 6 months of life with unusual and severe infections and severe failure to thrive. There is a profound defect of both cellular and humoral immunity (as the name implies).

**B** **True**

    **C**    **False**    These are more typical of chronic granulomatous disease, in which organisms are phagocytosed but not killed.

    **D**    **True**    Especially in male sibs, as some of this group are inherited as X-linked recessives.

    **E**    **False**

**I15**    **A**    **True**

    **B**    **True**

    **C**    **False**    A child of this age is still closely attached to parents and even the friendliest paediatric ward should not expect the child to tolerate admission for this long without parents.

    **D**    **False**

    **E**    **True**

**I16**    **A**    **True**    These children are at increased risk of both acute and chronic serous otitis media.

    **B**    **True**

    **C**    **False**    There is however an association with hypoparathyroidism, cardiac defects and immunodeficiency, which together constitute DiGeorge syndrome (or branchial arch syndrome). Recently this has been demonstrated to be due to a deletion on chromosome 22q11 (the so-called CATCH 22 syndrome).

    **D**    **True**    See (C)

    **E**    **True**    Micrognathia and a midline palatal cleft constitute the Pierre Robin syndrome.

**I17**    **A**    **True**    Raising the platelet count to higher levels reduces this risk, so commonsense dictates that it is reasonable to treat to reduce the risk of a potentially fatal complication. (Remarkably, some authorities prefer to wait until *after* the intracranial haemorrhage has occurred.) Treatment is with either steroids or immunoglobulins, both of which are effective. Platelet transfusions have such a brief effect that they are relatively useless.

    **B**    **False**    In childhood ITP, splenectomy is a last resort and is very rarely needed in the acute stages.

    **C**    **False**    ITP is due to increased rates of breakdown of platelets in the spleen due to antiplatelet antibodies.

**D** **False** Bone marrow examination is the recommended orthodoxy before *steroid* treatment because the latter can mask early leukaemia presenting as thrombocytopenia. However, the advantage of immunoglobulin is that it has no effect in masking leukaemia and so prior bone marrow examination is unnecessary.

**E** **True** The likelihood of remission is unaffected either way by treatment in the acute stages. However, this is *not* of itself an argument against treatment, see (A).

**I18** **A** **True** Like other causes of haemolytic disease of the newborn G6PD deficiency can cause severe neonatal jaundice which will be clinically apparent within the first 24 hours of life. Worldwide, this is the commonest diagnosis necessitating exchange transfusion.

**B** **False** Congenital hypothyroidism characteristically causes a prolongation of neonatal jaundice beyond 5–7 days, and does not normally cause jaundice in the first 24 hours.

**C** **True** Any severe congenital infection, whether viral or bacterial, can be expected to cause jaundice in the first 24 hours. However, most cases of congenital CMV infection are clinically normal at birth.

**D** **False** Choledochal cysts can cause obstructive jaundice, but this would not normally be apparent for several days.

**E** **False** While tyrosinaemia can present in severe form with jaundice and acute liver failure in infancy, it does not typically cause jaundice in the first 24 hours of life.

**I19** **A** **False** Reye syndrome is a rare condition characterized by encephalopathy, hypoglycaemia and convulsions. It carries a poor prognosis. There is evidence of hepatocellular dysfunction but jaundice is not a feature of the condition.

**B** **True** This follows official advice against the use of aspirin for febrile illnesses under the age of 12 years, after a statistical association was noted.

**C** **False** There is no specific treatment, and the management is basically supportive.

**D** **True** See (C).

**E** **True** Cerebral oedema may be a complication.

**I20    A    False**    DMSA is a radiopharmaceutical that is administered intravenously and extracted from the blood by the proximal tubules of the kidney where it is fixed. It renders the renal cortex radioactive so that the kidney parenchyme can be imaged. Very little isotope escapes into the urine. Other radio-isotope scans including DTPA and MAG3 can be used to follow the drainage of the urine.

**B    False**    Radio-isotope images of the kidney produce little anatomical detail of the collecting system but clearly reveal focal scarring of the cortex.

**C    False**    The radiation dose of a DMSA scan is low relative to alternatives such as the intravenous urogram (IVU), and the functional information obtained both in terms of focal scarring and renal activity is highly superior. This should be the first line of investigation for functional imaging.

**D    True**    DMSA scans are highly sensitive for areas of poor function. Damaged areas can be identified immediately, compared to the IVU where anatomical distortion is needed before scars can be readily identified, months or years later.

**E    True**    DMSA scans are highly sensitive and areas of reduced uptake due to renal inflammation may appear as a focal deficit that will disappear when the inflammation has settled. Unless the scan is delayed a further 8 weeks or so, false positive diagnoses of scarring will be made.

# PAPER J
## QUESTIONS

**J1** ***Staphylococcus pyogenes (aureus)* is the commonest causative organism in patients with:**
 A   neonatal meningitis.
 B   toxic epidermal necrolysis.
 C   mucocutaneous lymph node syndrome (Kawasaki disease).
 D   impetigo.
 E   hand, foot and mouth disease.

**J2** **With reference to the causation of abdominal pain:**
 A   the visceral peritoneum is insensitive to pain.
 B   appendicular spasm gives a pain referred to the right iliac fossa.
 C   pain due to stretching of smooth muscle fibres of the transverse colon is felt in the epigastrium.
 D   pain from obstruction to the pelviureteric junction typically radiates to the ipsilateral inguinal area.
 E   in herpes zoster of the abdominal wall, pain usually precedes the appearance of vesicles by several days.

**J3** **Recognized causes of intracranial calcification include:**
 A   histiocytosis X.
 B   craniopharyngioma.
 C   congenital toxoplasmosis.
 D   marble bone disease.
 E   Hurler syndrome.

**J4** **Cow's milk protein intolerance/allergy may present in the following ways:**
 A   bloody colitis in infancy.
 B   chronic wheezing in the first year of life.
 C   anaphylactic-like collapse.
 D   an exacerbation of eczema.
 E   infantile colic.

**J5** **The following are true concerning neonatal tetanus in the context of developing countries:**
 A   if the child survives he will be immune to tetanus.
 B   the shorter the incubation period the better the prognosis.

C   the condition can be prevented by active immunization of
    mothers against tetanus during the antenatal period.
D   benzylpenicillin is indicated.
E   the mortality rate is commonly over 40%.

**J6   Bronchopulmonary dysplasia (BPD):**
A   responds dramatically to tolazoline.
B   is more likely in infants who have received high-pressure
    mechanical ventilation.
C   may cause pulmonary hypertension.
D   usually resolves completely within 3 months if the infant
    survives.
E   involves destruction of alveoli.

**J7   Hypothermia can cause the following in low birth weight
       infants:**
A   decreased synthesis of surfactant.
B   hypernatraemia.
C   hypoglycaemia.
D   increased oxygen consumption.
E   hypercalcaemia.

**J8   The following statements are correct:**
A   total anomalous pulmonary venous drainage (TAPVD)
    typically produces pulmonary oligaemia.
B   aortic incompetence is a recognized feature of Marfan
    syndrome.
C   atrial septal defect (ASD) characteristically causes a
    pansystolic murmur.
D   children with aortic stenosis should not take strenuous
    exercise.
E   in children with congenital complete heart block the
    ventricular rate may increase with exercise.

**J9   In the management of diabetic ketoacidosis:**
A   rehydration is more important than insulin in the early
    stages.
B   it is not necessary to empty the stomach if there has been
    recent vomiting.
C   if the pretreatment potassium level is above 5 mmol/l no
    potassium should be given for the first 6 hours.
D   if the level of consciousness improves and then
    deteriorates despite orthodox treatment, the rate of
    intravenous fluids should be increased.
E   preceding dietary infringement is a likely precipitating
    cause of the ketoacidosis.

**J10   The following are characteristic findings in beta thalassaemia:**
A   hypochromic microcytic red cells.
B   low serum iron.

**C** cardiomyopathy.
**D** presentation in the neonatal period.
**E** frontal bossing of the skull.

**J11** **In juvenile rheumatoid arthritis:**
  **A** the pauciarticular type is least likely to suffer long-term disability.
  **B** the polyarticular type is more common in girls.
  **C** the systemic type carries the highest risk of iritis.
  **D** about 80% of children with iritis have a positive antinuclear factor.
  **E** the systemic type characteristically causes a polymorphonuclear leukocytosis.

**J12** **Characteristic features of idiopathic hypercalcaemia (severe type—Williams syndrome) include:**
  **A** diarrhoea.
  **B** supravalvar aortic stenosis.
  **C** elfin facies.
  **D** polyuria.
  **E** learning difficulties.

**J13** **In the case of a 2-year-old child brought to a casualty department with a fractured tibia, the following features are suggestive of non-accidental injury (NAI):**
  **A** a parental account that is precise, vivid and rich in detail.
  **B** bruising that appears older than the fracture.
  **C** parents who appear in a hurry to get away and leave their child in hospital.
  **D** delay in seeking medical attention.
  **E** a mother who seems upset and guilty about the 'accident' and keeps asking if the child will be all right.

**J14** **In the management of children with acute lymphatic leukaemia:**
  **A** oral sodium bicarbonate may be useful in the induction phase of treatment.
  **B** 6-mercaptopurine is one of the main drugs used in induction therapy.
  **C** vincristine is the drug of choice for intrathecal therapy in meningeal leukaemia.
  **D** prednisolone as low-dose continuous therapy is an orthodox part of long-term maintenance treatment.
  **E** the prognosis for girls is better than it is for boys.

**J15** **The following are characteristic features of infantile cortical hyperostosis (Caffey's disease):**
  **A** involvement of the spine.
  **B** dramatic response to steroid therapy.
  **C** raised erythrocyte sedimentation rate (ESR).

**D** lytic bone lesions on X-ray.
**E** commonest in early infancy.

**J16** **Down syndrome:**
**A** has a higher incidence of hypothyroidism than in normal children.
**B** occurs in approximately 1:2000 births.
**C** is associated with congenital heart disease in about 80% of cases.
**D** carries a significantly increased risk of epilepsy.
**E** may be due to translocation in about 6% of cases.

**J17** **In the assessment and investigation of a case of presumed idiopathic epilepsy:**
**A** computerized axial tomography is indicated in all cases under 14 years of age.
**B** it may be appropriate to examine both parents under Woods' (ultraviolet) light.
**C** if a random blood glucose is normal this precludes hypoglycaemia as a cause.
**D** if the EEG is abnormal this is an indication for treatment following a first convulsion.
**E** a history of rapid recovery of normal consciousness favours the diagnosis of a 'faint' rather than a 'fit'.

**J18** **In the clinical presentation of cerebral tumours in childhood:**
**A** tumours in the frontal region give early localizing signs.
**B** tumours in the parietal region typically present with early signs of raised intracranial pressure.
**C** posterior fossa tumours typically cause bitemporal hemianopia.
**D** medulloblastomas may cause truncal ataxia.
**E** episodic unilateral headache is a typical symptom of raised intracranial pressure.

**J19** **The following are recognized complications of cystic fibrosis:**
**A** proliferative glomerulonephritis.
**B** cirrhosis.
**C** heat exhaustion.
**D** diabetes mellitus.
**E** rectal prolapse.

**J20** **The following statements are true concerning rheumatic fever:**
**A** the risk of damage to heart valves is greatest in a first attack.
**B** following an attack, children should only receive penicillin prior to dental extractions.

**C**   steroid therapy during the acute attack does not affect the
     likelihood of permanent damage to heart valves.
**D**   the disease characteristically follows an infection with
     *Streptococcus viridans*.
**E**   presence of a mid-diastolic murmur at the apex during an
     attack suggests that a degree of subsequent mitral stenosis
     is inevitable.

# PAPER J
## ANSWERS

**J1** **A** **False** *Staphylococcus pyogenes* is an unusual cause of meningitis at any age, although it plays an important role in cerebral abscess. Neonatal meningitis is most commonly due to coliforms or the Group B streptococcus.

    **B** **True** Toxic epidermal necrolysis (Lyell's disease, Ritter's disease or the scalded skin syndrome) is a severe illness in which large areas of epidermis peel away from the inflamed dermis under the influence of a staphylococcal exotoxin. The child may look as if he/she has been scalded and in the absence of a history doctors may begin to consider the diagnosis of non-accidental injury. Nikolsky's sign is positive. Treatment consists of supportive measures plus eradication of the staphylococcus by systemic antibiotic therapy.

    **C** **False** Kawasaki disease is a rather bizarre multisystem disorder of as yet uncertain aetiology, although infection with a Rickettsia-like organism has been suggested. Staphylococcal infection plays no part in this illness.

    **D** **True** Impetigo is an infectious skin condition in which staphylococci are nearly always present. Streptococci may also be important in this condition. Pus from a lesion can lead to rapid involvement of previously normal skin. Topical antibiotic therapy may be sufficient if only a few lesions are present, otherwise systemic antibiotics are indicated.

    **E** **False** Hand, foot and mouth disease is a condition in which there is stomatitis together with vesicular lesions of the hands and feet. It is due to infection with Coxsackie A virus, usually the A 16 strain.

**J2** **A** **True** The visceral peritoneum, pericardium and pleura are insensitive to pain, whereas their parietal portions are sensitive to pain, being supplied with sensory nerve fibres which travel along peripheral nerves.

**B   False**   Pain due to appendicular colic is referred to the midline, as is the case with all unpaired viscera, and it is felt at the level of the umbilicus, whereas small bowel colic is felt in the epigastrium, and large bowel colic is felt in the hypogastrium. In acute appendicitis, pain eventually is felt in the right iliac fossa but this is due to inflammation of parietal peritoneum, and is dull and constant rather than colicky.

**C   False**   The site of referral of pain due to gut colic is unrelated to the anatomical position of the portion of gut concerned. As already stated, large gut colic — whether ascending, transverse or descending colon — is referred to the hypogastrium in the midline.

**D   False**   Ureteric colic is characteristically felt down one side of the anterior abdominal wall radiating to the groin. Pain due to distension of the capsule of the kidney is typically felt in the loin and upper abdomen. In pelviureteric junction obstruction, there is no reason for pain to arise from the lower ureter and pain is not likely to be felt in the inguinal area.

**E   True**   Pain due to herpes zoster infection (shingles) usually precedes the appearance of vesicles by several days, and this can lead to it simulating an acute abdomen.

**J3   A   False**   The histiocytosis X group of conditions comprises a spectrum of increasing severity with reducing age. The mildest form, which occurs in older children, is eosinophilic granuloma, which consists of single or multiple osteolytic lesions. The next variety is Hand–Schüller–Christian disease with multiple lytic bony lesions especially involving the skull, diabetes insipidus, pulmonary infiltration and proptosis. The rarest and most severe variety is Letterer–Siwe disease which has all the above plus skin involvement and hepatosplenomegaly. None of these conditions gives intracranial calcification.

**B   True**   Craniopharyngioma is the commonest pituitary tumour in childhood, and may present with raised intracranial pressure, visual impairment or growth failure. Diabetes insipidus may also occur, together with features of hypopituitarism. Lateral skull X-ray characteristically shows calcification in the suprasellar region with possible enlargement of the pituitary fossa.

**C** **True** Congenital toxoplasmosis may cause choroidoretinitis, microcephaly, severe retardation and later epilepsy. It also causes intracranial calcification.

**D** **False** Marble bone disease is a condition in which the entire skeleton is sclerotic, the bones are dense but fragile and the marrow cavity is encroached upon. In the severe recessive form there is a poor prognosis due to pancytopenia leading to haemorrhage, anaemia and recurrent infections. The more benign form is inherited as a dominant and is compatible with a normal lifespan. Neither form causes intracranial calcification.

**E** **False** Hurler syndrome (gargoylism) is not a recognized cause of intracranial calcification.

**J4** **A** **True** It is possible that cow's milk intolerance is the commonest cause of 'colitis' in infancy. Simple trial of exclusion followed by challenge is the most useful approach to diagnosis, as results of other investigations may be conflicting or unhelpful. Cases have been described where this syndrome occurred in breastfed infants and was cured by the mother excluding cow's milk from her diet.

**B** **True** Again, a trial of dietary exclusion, followed if appropriate by challenge, is the best approach to diagnosis. Some of these children may be early cases of asthma.

**C** **True** Infants may suffer a life-threatening anaphylactic-like collapse on exposure to cow's milk protein. This is almost certainly a true Type I immediate hypersensitivity reaction. It may appear to occur on first exposure, e.g. at 4 months in a mother who has initially breast fed. In these cases presumably sensitization has occurred earlier by prior exposure, e.g. on a postnatal ward. These children should *not* be challenged until they are much older because of the dangers involved.

**D** **True** The aetiology of eczema is complex and multifactorial and the role of cow's milk allergy is still the subject of some controversy. However, atopic infants frequently develop an exacerbation of eczema on exposure to cow's milk protein and are helped by exclusion.

**E   True**   A significant proportion of 'colicky' infants are helped by exclusion of cow's milk protein from their diets, or from the diets of their breast feeding mothers, and will relapse on re-exposure. Prior to this observation, 3-month colic had been regarded as almost totally a psychosomatic disease.

**J5   A   False**   Neither neonatal tetanus nor tetanus in later life conveys immunity to the disease. This is a reflection of the extremely small quantity of toxin needed to produce the disease.

**B   False**   A short incubation period carries a worse prognosis.

**C   True**   If the mother has already been actively immunized in childhood a booster dose will suffice. A preventive policy is likely to be highly cost-effective.

**D   True**   While penicillin has no action on the neurotoxin, it can eradicate the tetanus bacilli and prevent synthesis of further toxin.

**E   True**   Even fully developed intensive care facilities are unlikely to improve the mortality very significantly, and such facilities are extremely unlikely to be widely available in the short-term future.

**J6   A   False**   Tolazoline is not effective in the management of bronchopulmonary dysplasia. It is mainly used in severe hyaline membrane disease and persistent fetal circulation, because of its action as a pulmonary vasodilator.

**B   True**   High ventilatory pressures for prolonged periods are probably the most important cause of BPD and the disease is very unusual in infants who have not received IPPV. Other contributory factors are thought to include oxygen toxicity, infection and the presence of an endotracheal tube interfering with clearing of secretions.

**C   True**   Pathologically there is widespread peribronchiolar fibroplasia with areas of collapse and compensatory emphysema. Pulmonary hypertension and cor pulmonale may develop and prove fatal.

**D   False**   Severe cases of BPD who survive may have significantly abnormal blood gases for the first year of life and these gradually return to normal as the alveoli regenerate.

**E   True**

**J7** **A** **True** Hypothermia directly reduces the synthesis of surfactant. It may also have the same effect indirectly by causing acidosis. Avoiding cooling of preterm neonates significantly reduces the risk of subsequent development of hyaline membrane disease.

**B** **False** Hypothermia is not a recognized cause of hypernatraemia whereas hyperpyrexia is, through increased fluid loss by evaporation and sweating.

**C** **True** Hypothermia leads to an increased metabolic stress on the neonate in its efforts to maintain body temperature. Depletion of glycogen stores, hypoglycaemia and acidosis all occur.

**D** **True** Moderate hypothermia leads to increased oxygen consumption. Prolonged or severe hypothermia (core temperature below 32°C) leads to reduced oxygen consumption.

**E** **False**

**J8** **A** **False** In TAPVD the pulmonary veins return to the right atrium instead of the left. This increases the volume of blood on the right side of the heart, and therefore through the lungs. There is therefore pulmonary plethora rather than oligaemia.

**B** **True** Dissecting aneurysm is also a complication. The pulmonary artery may be affected in a similar fashion.

**C** **False** The typical murmur of ASD is an ejection systolic murmur in the pulmonary area. There are only three conditions which give pansystolic murmurs: ventricular septal defect, mitral incompetence and tricuspid incompetence.

**D.** **True** This is because of the risk of sudden death.

**E** **True** This contrasts with acquired complete heart block in adults where there is no increase in rate with exercise.

**J9** **A** **True** Hypovolaemic circulatory failure compounded by metabolic acidosis is the most likely early cause of death. Hyperglycaemia by itself is relatively harmless. Rapid reversal of circulatory failure is therefore the most important early priority, although naturally insulin is given as well in the initial stages.

**B  False**  Considerable gastric atony is common in diabetic ketoacidosis and one vomit may not have emptied the stomach completely. There will thus be a continued risk of vomiting and aspiration in the seriously ill patient, and so it is wise to empty the stomach in such cases and leave an indwelling nasogastric tube on free drainage.

**C  False**  Virtually all patients with ketoacidosis are significantly depleted of total body potassium. High pretreatment serum levels are common but misleading, being due to the severe metabolic acidosis causing a shift of intracellular potassium into the extracellular fluid. The initial potassium depletion, followed by rapid rehydration with 0.9% saline, together with what is in effect 'glucose and insulin treatment' all constitute a potent recipe for hypokalaemia within the first 4 hours. It is therefore reasonable to ignore the initial potassium level and to start intravenous potassium supplementation at around 4 hours, after the initial period of rapid rehydration.

**D  False**  The deterioration is likely to be due to cerebral oedema, which is a rare but extremely serious complication which carries a high risk of death or brain damage. Management consists of urgent restriction of fluids together with mannitol and elective ventilation. This complication may be more common since the advent of continuous low-dose insulin regimens; it is possible that these are so effective at lowering blood sugar that too early recourse is being made to fluids such as 4% dextrose in 0.18% saline, and that such fluids, if given at faster than maintenance rates, could contribute to cerebral oedema.

**E  False**  Dietary infringements with excess calorie intake should only lead to hyperglycaemia and glycosuria. As long as the normal insulin is given there should be no ketoacidosis. The most likely cause of ketoacidosis occurring despite normal insulin therapy is intercurrent infection.

**J10  A  True**  This is a reflection of the defective synthesis of haemoglobin in this condition.

**B** **False** As with other chronic haemolytic anaemias, the serum iron is raised. This problem is worse in thalassaemia because of the necessity for multiple transfusions, and the transfusional haemosiderosis is the main cause of mortality in treated children. Attempts to lessen the iron overload with continuous subcutaneous infusions of desferrioxamine are being made. The skin of a child with haemosiderosis is typically slate grey, due to the increased deposition of both iron and melanin.

**C** **True** The cardiomyopathy is secondary to iron overload and is one of the main causes of mortality. It leads to heart failure and arrhythmias which may both be very refractory to drug treatment. Iron overload also causes cirrhosis of the liver.

**D** **False** Fetal haemoglobin is the predominant haemoglobin type at birth. Infants with thalassaemia are usually significantly anaemic by the age of 6 months.

**E** **True** This is also a feature of sickle cell disease, and in both conditions is due to marrow hyperplasia. The skull X-ray in both conditions is described as showing a 'hair-on-end' appearance.

**J11** **A** **True** Apart from the 25% risk of iritis, the pauciarticular form is the best to have, as long-term severe disability is rare in this condition.

**B** **True** About 80% of patients are girls. This variety carries a 15% risk of severe disability.

**C** **False** There is virtually no risk of iritis in the systemic type.

**D** **True**

**E** **True**

**J12** **A** **False** Hypercalcaemia at any age tends to cause constipation not diarrhoea. As the severe form of this condition causes mental retardation, there is a danger that a child may be regarded as having idiopathic retardation with constipation as a secondary symptom. Measurement of serum calcium should always be included in the investigation of unexplained psychomotor retardation, especially as this is one of the few treatable causes of retardation.

**B** **True** Either aortic or pulmonary stenosis may occur in idiopathic hypercalcaemia, and these are usually of the supravalvar variety.

**C** **True** Most cases of the more severe variety of idiopathic hypercalcaemia have abnormal facies usually described as 'elfin'. The lips are prominent with a short up-turned nose with a flattened bridge. Hypertelorism and low-set prominent ears are also present with prominent cheeks.

**D** **True** Hypercalcaemia causes renal damage and can progress to nephrocalcinosis and chronic renal failure. Tubular damage is greater than that to glomeruli, so loss of concentrating power is a prominent feature. This results in polyuria and polydipsia.

**E** **True** Children with abnormal facies usually have significant learning difficulties.

**J13** **A** **False** In most cases of NAI the parents are forced to invent a plausible account. These accounts are usually rather vague and lacking in detail. In contrast, a parent whose child has had a genuine accident can usually give a very detailed story which carries conviction. However there is no certainty in this difficult area and an exception to the above statements can exist when parents have the time and presence of mind to invent a really good story.

**B** **True** Injuries of different ages should always suggest the diagnosis of NAI in children as young as this. Again they are not utterly diagnostic, but this is an area where the most important step in diagnosis is to think of it in the first place.

**C** **True** This is highly suggestive of NAI, as if the parents do not wish to be questioned too closely. The willingness to leave a child this age alone in hospital is unnatural and suggests defective parent-child bonding.

**D** **True** Again this is a strong pointer to NAI, as if the parents were hoping that the injury would go away. Prompt seeking of medical help does not exclude the diagnosis of NAI.

**E** **False** This is natural behaviour for a normal 'creatively anxious' mother whose child has had an injury of this severity. Absence of this behaviour would be grounds for concern. Of course, it could be normal behaviour for an innocent mother whose cohabitee had caused the fracture, but such a mother would be unlikely to conceal the truth for long.

**J14**  **A**  **True**  One of the hazards of induction therapy is hyperuricaemia with uricosuria, which may result in crystalluria and obstructive renal failure. This risk can be minimized by (1) liberal fluid intake, (2) alkalinizing the urine with oral sodium bicarbonate, and (3) use of allopurinol, which inhibits xanthine oxidase, thus impairing the synthesis of uric acid.

  **B**  **False**  The drugs most commonly used in induction therapy are vincristine, prednisolone and L-asparaginase. 6-mercaptopurine is used in maintenance therapy.

  **C**  **False**  Methotrexate is the drug of choice for intrathecal therapy, for which vincristine is totally unsuitable, as it is potentially lethal by this route.

  **D**  **False**  Prednisolone is used in high doses in induction-phase treatment, and in recurrent monthly 5-day pulses throughout maintenance treatment. Other drugs (6-mercaptopurine and methotrexate) are preferred for continuous maintenance therapy.

  **E**  **True**  In addition to being male, other poor prognostic factors include a high white cell count at diagnosis and the presence of a mediastinal mass.

**J15**  **A**  **False**  Caffey's disease, which is of unknown aetiology, may affect the flat bones, including the mandible, scapulae, ilium and frontal and parietal bones. It may also affect long bones but spares the spine. It presents with fever, irritability and soft tissue swellings. X-rays show subperiosteal new bone formation which may lead to a mistaken diagnosis of non-accidental injury. ESR and platelet count are typically elevated.

  **B**  **True**  Steroids are very effective at reducing fever and systemic upset.

  **C**  **True**

  **D**  **False**  There is no lysis of bone, only subperiosteal new bone formation.

  **E**  **True**  The condition almost invariably starts within the first 5 months of life.

**J16**  **A**  **True**  As both Down syndrome and hypothyroidism cause short stature and mental retardation, it is rather easy to miss the diagnosis of hypothyroidism when it occurs in a child with Down syndrome.

**B    False**    The overall incidence of Down syndrome is about 1:600 births. The incidence rises with increasing maternal age over 35 years, and is about 1:200 in mothers aged 40 years.

**C    False**    The incidence of congenital heart disease is approximately 20% and ventricular septal defect is the commonest lesion.

**D    False**

**E    True**    Cases of Down syndrome due to translocation occur at any maternal age. Both the parents should have their chromosomes studied and more extended family studies should be done as necessary.

**J17    A    False**    CT (or MRI) scanning should be reserved for cases of focal epilepsy or those with clinical evidence of neurological deficit.

**B    True**    If the child has hypopigmented areas of skin, the possibility of tuberous sclerosis should be considered. As this is inherited as a dominant condition, finding some of the features in one parent will strengthen the diagnosis.

**C    False**    A normal random blood glucose cannot prove anything. If hypoglycaemia is to be excluded, a fasting blood sugar is the investigation required.

**D    False**    An abnormal EEG would not override the basic rule that anticonvulsants are only proffered after a *second* convulsion.

**E    True**    In a vasovagal faint, consciousness is lost because of decreased cerebral blood flow. Once the latter returns to normal, consciousness is regained rapidly. In contrast, an epileptiform attack is characteristically followed by a period of disturbed consciousness.

**J18    A    False**    The frontal region is a 'silent' area of the brain in terms of localizing signs. As a result, frontal lobe tumours are usually detected late. Personality change or intellectual deterioration may be the first abnormal symptom.

**B    False**    Most tumours that cause early raised intracranial pressure do so by obstruction of CSF pathways, most commonly tumours in the posterior fossa. Parietal tumours can only cause raised intracranial pressure by very rapid growth, and in this case even earlier presentation with epilepsy or hemiplegia would be likely.

**C**   **False**   As already stated, posterior fossa tumours typically cause early raised intracranial pressure. They cannot cause visual field defects of any kind. The only cause of bitemporal hemianopia is a lesion of the optic chiasm, and the commonest cause of this in childhood is a craniopharyngioma.

**D**   **True**   Medulloblastomas are the commonest cerebral tumours in childhood, accounting for 50% of all such tumours. They nearly always arise in the vermis of the cerebellum, and grow out to involve the cerebellar hemispheres. They are the only cerebral tumours to metastasize, and do so via CSF pathways. They usually present with signs of raised intracranial pressure, but a possible earlier presentation is with unsteadiness of gait without necessarily any cerebellar signs in the limbs (truncal ataxia). This may easily be dismissed as hysterical in origin.

**E**   **False**   Raised intracranial pressure typically is present on waking and gradually improves during the day. It is not lateralized and is felt worse in the frontal region. It is not episodic as it is present for most of every day. Most episodic unilateral headaches with a throbbing character are due to migraine.

**J19**   **A**   **False**

**B**   **True**   Cirrhosis is a relatively late complication of cystic fibrosis, and is of the biliary type, due to obstruction of bile ductules by viscid secretions.

**C**   **True**   Because of the high sodium content of sweat, children with cystic fibrosis are at risk of heat exhaustion (sodium depletion) during hot summers or when living in the tropics. This phenomenon was first noted during a heat wave in New York. It can be prevented by salt supplements.

**D**   **True**   Again this is a late complication and is due to involvement of the islets of Langerhans by the pancreatic damage basic to this condition.

**E**   **True**   Rectal prolapse is quite a common symptom in children with cystic fibrosis, especially during the first 3 years of life.

**J20**   **A**   **False**   The heart may escape any long-term complications in a first attack and the risk of these developing is considerably greater in second and subsequent attacks. This emphasizes the vital nature of effective long-term penicillin prophylaxis, which should be given *continuously* for 10–15 years after a first attack.

**B   False**   See (A). Prophylaxis to cover dental extractions is a different issue, and is aimed at the prevention of bacterial endocarditis in children with established structural cardiac defects, either congenital or acquired.

**C   True**   Steroid therapy is, however, justified in the short term as it has a significant effect on diminishing symptoms.

**D   False**   *Streptococcus viridans* is a common causative organism in subacute bacterial endocarditis but does not cause rheumatic fever. Rheumatic fever is precipitated by any β-haemolytic streptococcal infection, usually tonsillitis.

**E   False**   Such a murmur (the Carey Coombs murmur) may commonly be heard in a first attack from which the heart may emerge unscathed. It is thought to be due to transient valvulitis of the mitral valve.

# PAPER K
## QUESTIONS

K1 The following conditions should be suspected in a 3-week-old breast feeding infant who is jaundiced and has a total bilirubin of 156 µmol/l (of which 70 µmol/l is conjugated), an aspartate aminotransferase (AST) level of 140 i.u./l and an alkaline phosphatase activity of 502 i.u./l:

    A   breast milk jaundice.
    B   neonatal hepatitis.
    C   hypothyroidism.
    D   galactosaemia.
    E   phenylketonuria.

K2 The following statements are true concerning the mechanism of action of drugs used in the treatment of asthma:

    A   aminophylline leads to regeneration of cyclic adenine monophosphate (AMP) in bronchial smooth muscle.
    B   steroid therapy has the effect of restoring the responsiveness of bronchi to bronchodilators.
    C   bronchodilators can lead to a reduction in arterial $Po_2$ despite symptomatic improvement.
    D   inhaled beclomethasone needs to be taken four times a day for full protective effect.
    E   oral prednisolone takes 24 hours to produce a detectable improvement in an acute attack.

K3 The following are recognized features of infections with viruses of the Coxsackie group:

    A   epidemic pleurodynia (Bornholm disease).
    B   herpangina.
    C   parotitis.
    D   erythema nodosum.
    E   hand, foot and mouth disease.

K4 The following conditions have a recognized association with erythema nodosum:

    A   Crohn's disease.
    B   cat-scratch fever.
    C   roseola infantum.
    D   lepromatous leprosy.
    E   molluscum contagiosum.

**K5  In the management of burns in childhood:**
A  blisters should be pricked prior to transport to hospital.
B  narcotic analgesics should be avoided.
C  children with burns affecting more than 10% of their body area should have an intravenous line set up.
D  the child's status with respect to immunity to tetanus should be ascertained.
E  early elective endotracheal intubation is indicated if the face and neck have been involved in the burn.

**K6  In tuberculous meningitis in childhood:**
A  the Mantoux reaction is negative.
B  the CSF glucose level is characteristically reduced.
C  the CSF reaction consists mainly of polymorphs.
D  the presentation is characteristically subacute.
E  rifampicin is not a useful drug for treating this condition.

**K7  The following substances are freely transmitted across the placenta:**
A  carbimazole.
B  diazepam.
C  warfarin.
D  pethidine.
E  IgM antibodies.

**K8  In the normal newborn infant in the first 24 hours of life:**
A  many significant heart defects may be clinically undetectable.
B  a normal arterial $po_2$ helps the ductus to close.
C  hypoxia causes pulmonary artery vasoconstriction.
D  all children with murmurs heard in the first 24 hours should be followed up for at least 6 months.
E  the systolic blood pressure is between 40 and 80 mmHg.

**K9  Infantile hypertrophic pyloric stenosis:**
A  characteristically presents between 3 and 6 months of age.
B  typically presents with a sodium of c. 110 mmol/l.
C  causes a hypokalaemic alkalosis.
D  is commoner in female than in male infants.
E  has a significant familial tendency.

**K10  In the management of growth disorders in childhood:**
A  all 2-year-old children below the 3rd centile for weight should have a jejunal biopsy to exclude coeliac disease.
B  growth hormone deficiency seldom presents with poor growth until the 2nd and 3rd years of life.
C  maximal increase in head circumference occurs in the 2nd year of life.
D  absence of symptoms coupled with a normal xylose tolerance test excludes coeliac disease.

**E** if obesity is due to Cushing syndrome the height is also usually above average.

**K11** **Concerning neuroblastoma in childhood:**
**A** the primary tumour is intra-abdominal in over 50% of cases.
**B** the prospect for cure in children presenting with metastatic disease is less than 30%.
**C** intra-abdominal tumours rarely cross the midline.
**D** straight abdominal X-ray may show calcification within the tumour mass.
**E** raised urinary levels of vanillylmandelic acid (VMA) are a characteristic finding.

**K12** **The management of chronic renal failure in young children typically includes the following therapies:**
**A** calcium carbonate.
**B** erythropoietin.
**C** growth hormone.
**D** gastrostomy feeding.
**E** 1 $\alpha$-hydroxy vitamin $D_3$.

**K13** **The following statements are true concerning Type I glycogen storage disease (von Gierke's disease):**
**A** the prognosis is better than that in glycogen storage disease Type III.
**B** cardiomyopathy is a prominent feature of the disease.
**C** hyperuricaemia is a recognized feature of the disease.
**D** the kidneys may be enlarged and palpable.
**E** myoglobinuria may occur after exercise.

**K14** **The following are recognized features of Noonan syndrome (Bonnevie–Ulrich syndrome):**
**A** webbing of the neck.
**B** oedema in the neonatal period.
**C** 45 X karyotype.
**D** pulmonary stenosis.
**E** polycystic kidneys.

**K15** **The following statements are true with respect to viral encephalitis:**
**A** subacute sclerosing panencephalitis (SSPE) is thought to be due to mumps virus.
**B** focal signs are common in herpes simplex encephalitis.
**C** measles encephalitis characteristically affects the cerebellum.
**D** encephalitis occurs in about 1:1000 cases of measles.
**E** brain biopsy can confirm the diagnosis in herpes simplex encephalitis.

**K16    In the Guillain–Barré syndrome in childhood:**
A   a degree of permanent paralysis is characteristic.
B   increased reflexes in the lower limbs are characteristic.
C   paraesthesiae are characteristic.
D   the CSF protein concentration is elevated.
E   involvement of the autonomic nervous system is a recognized complication.

**K17    The following conditions are characteristically inherited as autosomal recessives:**
A   tuberous sclerosis.
B   galactosaemia.
C   pseudohypertrophic (Duchenne) muscular dystrophy.
D   cystic fibrosis.
E   chronic granulomatous disease of childhood.

**K18    Perthes' disease of the hip:**
A   is commoner in girls than in boys.
B   characteristically causes a raised ESR.
C   may cause wasting of the gluteal muscles.
D   may be excluded by a normal straight X-ray of the hip joint.
E   characteristically occurs in children over the age of 10 years.

**K19    Concerning brain growth, development and function in infancy:**
A   maximal neuronal proliferation occurs in the 3rd trimester of pregnancy.
B   the newborn brain is less susceptible than the adult brain to the effects of hypoxia.
C   head circumference increases in linear fashion over the first 2 years of life.
D   the main changes in the brain over the age from 0 to 2 years are myelination and glial proliferation.
E   convulsions can present in the newborn as apnoeic attacks.

**K20    The following can cause hypokalaemia:**
A   intravenous hydrocortisone.
B   acute haemolysis.
C   oral theophylline.
D   metabolic acidosis.
E   Bartter syndrome.

# PAPER K
## ANSWERS

**K1**

**A** **False** Breast milk jaundice is characterized by raised unconjugated bilirubin, possibly due to competitive inhibition of hepatic glucuronyl transferase by a steroid in breast milk. This diagnosis cannot explain the above laboratory findings which show evidence of both hepatitis (raised AST) and obstruction (raised alkaline phosphatase).

**B** **True** The above findings could be due to either neonatal hepatitis or biliary atresia, two serious conditions between which it is almost impossible to differentiate on clinical or laboratory evidence. Possible causes of neonatal hepatitis include congenital infection, e.g. rubella, cytomegalovirus and toxoplasmosis, and metabolic causes such as $\alpha_1$-antitrypsin deficiency and galactosaemia.

**C** **False** Congenital hypothyroidism should always be considered in prolonged neonatal jaundice. However, like breast milk jaundice it will cause an unconjugated hyperbilirubinaemia without evidence of hepatitis or obstruction.

**D** **True** Galactosaemia is an important (because treatable) but rare cause of neonatal hepatitis. The urine will give a positive reaction with Clinitest tablets, as galactose is a reducing substance.

**E** **False** Phenylketonuria is not a cause of prolonged neonatal jaundice.

**K2    A    True**

    **B    True**    Steriods do have other effects, e.g. reducing the inflammatory response and decreasing mucosal oedema.

    **C    True**    This fact is thought to be part of the explanation for the epidemic of asthma deaths in the 1960s. The theoretical explanation for this observed reduction of $PaO_2$ is as follows. In an attack of asthma some alveoli are underventilated. Reflex vasoconstriction of the pulmonary arteriole supplying these areas tends to compensate for this and to reduce right-to-left shunting. Virtually all bronchodilators are also pulmonary vasodilators and this can abolish this compensatory vasoconstriction. If the alveoli remain collapsed due to proximal mucosal oedema and mucus plugging there will be increased shunting and reduced arterial $PO_2$ despite bronchodilatation and symptomatic improvement. This mechanism constitutes strong justification for the use of short courses of steroids in acute attacks rather than relying solely on bronchodilators.

    **D    False**    Beclomethasone has a relatively long duration of action and can be fully effective taken twice a day.

    **E    False**    Oral prednisolone probably begins to produce significant effects within 3 hours of commencement of a course.

**K3    A    True**    This striking clinical condition is due to infection with certain group B Coxsackie viruses. It is characterized by a febrile illness followed by severe pain in the chest or abdomen simulating pleurisy or an acute abdomen. The pain probably originates from muscles of the chest or abdominal walls, and tenderness may be elicited on palpation. Diaphragmatic involvement may give referred pain in the supraclavicular area.

    **B    True**    Herpangina is a clear-cut clinical syndrome due to infection with Group A Coxsackie viruses. The characteristic feature is of five to six papulovesicular lesions around the tonsillar area and on the soft palate.

    **C    False**

    **D    False**

**E** **True** This condition consists of vesicular eruptions on the fingers and toes associated with a mild stomatitis with vesicular or ulcerated lesions on the tongue. It is thought to be due to infection with Coxsackie A viruses, usually A16.

In addition to the above, Coxsackie B viruses cause aseptic meningitis, encephalitis, a polio-like illness, pericarditis and myocarditis.

**K4** **A** **True** Erythema nodosum may occur in both Crohn's disease and ulcerative colitis. It may antedate the onset of symptoms attributable to bowel disease.

**B** **True** This benign illness is thought to be caused by a bacillus (*Rochalimaea henselae*) and consists of a febrile illness with malaise and lymphadenopathy. In about one third of cases there is suppuration of lymph glands. The infection is thought to be transmitted in cat saliva. Erythema nodosum is a recognized association.

**C** **False** The rash in this condition affects both trunk and limbs and is maculopapular in nature. The rash typically occurs on the fourth day of a feverish illness just as the fever is about to resolve. This condition is caused by parvovirus B19.

**D** **True** Erythema nodosum can be a troublesome complication of lepromatous leprosy and usually occurs after chemotherapy has been instituted.

**E** **False**

**K5** **A** **False** Even dead skin is a barrier to infection, and should certainly not be discarded at this early stage.

**B** **False** A child with moderate to severe burns is likely to experience both pain and fear and narcotic analgesics are the best treatment for both. Good analgesia will help to lessen the neurogenic component of shock.

**C** **True** A child with more than 10% burns is likely to lose significant quantities of extracellular fluid and plasma from the burnt surface and these may need to be replaced intravenously. Transfusions of both blood and plasma are likely to be essential with more extensive burns.

**D** **True** A necrotic area of burnt tissue is a potential site for the multiplication of tetanus bacilli, and tetanus prophylaxis is just as important for burns cases as it is for those with penetrating wounds. Prophylactic penicillin is advisable in the non-immune patient.

**E  True**   Burns involving the face and neck may lead to gross soft tissue swelling, which may make subsequent attempts to secure an airway very difficult.

**K6  A  False**   The Mantoux reaction will usually be strongly positive except in cases which are so advanced as to be virtually moribund.

**B  True**   In the early stages the CSF glucose may be normal and the cellular reaction a mixture of polymorphs and lymphocytes. However, in most cases by the time of diagnosis the CSF glucose will have fallen and the cellular reaction will be mainly lymphocytic. Compared with cases of viral meningitis the patient will be more ill, the onset more subacute, and the CSF protein higher, in addition to the low CSF glucose. If choroidal tubercles are present they are virtually diagnostic.

**C  False**   See (B).

**D  True**   For the first week or two of the illness the main symptoms are usually very non-specific, consisting of malaise, anorexia, lethargy and weight loss, with the subsequent development of headache, vomiting and drowsiness. Late diagnosis is the main reason for children dying or suffering brain damage from this condition.

**E  False**   Rifampicin and isoniazid are probably the main drugs to be used in this condition, with the possible addition of either ethambutol or streptomycin. Systemic or intrathecal steroid therapy may be indicated for the prevention and treatment of meningeal adhesions and spinal block. Prophylactic anticonvulsant medication, for example phenobarbitone, is advisable.

**K7  A  True**   Carbimazole administered to a thyrotoxic mother during pregnancy will enter the fetal circulation and can result in a goitre in the neonate.

**B  True**   Diazepam given to a pregnant woman, either in high-dose boluses close to delivery or low-dose long-term therapy in the last trimester, can produce profoundly affected infants with respiratory depression, hypotonia, feeding difficulties and poor temperature control.

**C  True**   Warfarin crosses the placenta and can cause a coagulation disorder in the neonate which should be preventable by prompt use of vitamin K. If used in early pregnancy, warfarin causes a condition similar to chondrodysplasia punctata in the infant.

**D** **True** Pethidine given as an analgesic in labour is a common cause of respiratory depression post delivery. This is more likely to result if the pethidine is given 4 hours before delivery than if it is given just before delivery. Naloxone is used to reverse the effects of pethidine.

**E** **False** IgM antibodies do not cross the placenta as their molecular weight is too high. Thus naturally occurring anti-A and anti-B do not cross the placenta as they are IgM antibodies. IgG antibodies do cross the placenta freely, and are a source of passive immunity for the infant, diminishing over the first 6 months of life.

**K8** **A** **True** For example, ventricular septal defects of moderate size may produce no murmurs because there is little left-to-right flow, due to the fact that the pulmonary vascular resistance has not yet fallen to normal limits. Another example is preductal coarctation of the aorta where the ductus arteriosus remains open allowing significant flow to the lower extremities; when the duct closes at around the end of the first week of life this can produce severe unexpected left-sided failure of rapid onset.

**B** **True** Conversely hypoxia favours the duct remaining patent, especially in preterm infants.

**C** **True**

**D** **False** The majority of murmurs heard in the first 24 hours of life are either functional or due to transient patency of the ductus arteriosus. If these murmurs are absent on the day of discharge from hospital there is no indication for special follow-up. However, all infants should be checked for murmurs in the community at the 6-week check.

**E** **True**

**K9** **A** **False** This condition usually presents between the ages of 3 and 6 *weeks* of age.

**B** **False** A 3-week-old vomiting infant with a sodium as low as this is more likely to be suffering from congenital adrenal hyperplasia.

**C** **True** The repeated vomiting leads to loss of $H^+$, $Na^+$, $K^+$ ions and, of course, water. The loss of $H^+$ and $K^+$ ions leads to alkalosis and hypokalaemia respectively. Renal compensation for the alkalosis leads to further potassium loss in an attempt to conserve $H^+$, and this aggravates the hypokalaemia.

**D** **False** Pyloric stenosis is commoner in male infants, the ratio to females being approximately five to one.

**E** **True** Pyloric stenosis has a tendency to run in families, inheritance probably being polygenic.

**K10** **A** **False** Three out of every 100 normal children are entitled to have a weight below the 3rd centile. Many others are entitled to lose weight to this extent after an acute illness such as measles or gastroenteritis. To subject all these children to jejunal biopsy would be quite unreasonable. In reaching decisions to investigate, far more attention should be paid to *serial* measurements and to evidence of fall-off through centile lines. See also (D) below.

**B** **True** Severe growth hormone deficiency from birth may present with hypoglycaemia in the first year of life, but growth failure from this cause is usually not recognized till the second year of life.

**C** **False** Maximal increase in head circumference occurs in the first year of life, and most of this is in the first 6 months. The average child's head grows by 9 cm in the first 6 months, 11 cm in the first 12 months and grows only 6 cm in the next 17 years. All this increase is due not to neuronal proliferation but to increasing differentiation of existing neurons together with glial proliferation.

**D** **False** Neither absence of symptoms nor a normal xylose tolerance test can exclude coeliac disease. Whereas the definitive investigation is still repeated jejunal biopsies, the measurement of endomyseal antibodies is a very useful first-line screening investigation.

**E** **False** The obesity of Cushing syndrome is due to excessive steroid secretion, and is classically of the 'pear-on-matchsticks' variety. Additional features include buffalo hump and striae. The effect of steroids on the epiphyses is to stunt growth so children with Cushing syndrome will tend to have heights below average with evidence of fall-off since the onset of the condition. The far more common condition of simple obesity is usually associated with above-average height, and this is a useful distinction in clinical practice.

**K11** **A** **True** Most cases arise from the adrenal medulla or retroperitoneal sympathetic ganglia. Some tumours originate in sympathetic ganglia of the neck, thorax or pelvis.

**B** **True**

**C** **False**  In this respect it tends to differ from nephroblastoma which tends not to cross the midline.

**D** **True**

**E** **True**  These are present in over 90% of affected children.

**K12** **A** **True**  Calcium carbonate administered around meal times binds with the dietary phosphate to render it non-absorbable and thereby lowers the plasma phosphate. Avoiding hyperphosphataemia prevents the suppression of 1 $\alpha$-hydroxylation of Vitamin D and protects against renal rickets.

**B** **True**  Now available as a recombinant product, erythropoietin has been shown to be of value in children with renal failure by producing a better quality of life through avoidance of anaemia and by preventing the need for repeated blood transfusions.

**C** **True**  Growth hormone has been conclusively shown to be of value in children with poor growth due to chronic renal failure and is now used extensively.

**D** **True**  Young infants and children with chronic renal failure have a poorly understood anorexia which leads to failure to thrive. In these cases good nutrition can often be adequately provided only by nasogastric tube or gastrostomy feeding.

**E** **True**  1$\alpha$-hydroxylation occurs in the proximal tubule cells, and in children with chronic renal failure little 1 $\alpha$-hydroxylation occurs.

**K13** **A** **False**  Type I and Type III are clinically similar, presenting with hepatomegaly, hypoglycaemia, short stature and doll-like facies. However, Type III is the milder disease with a less severe tendency to hypoglycaemia.

**B** **False**  Cardiomyopathy is a feature of Type II disease (Pompe's disease).

**C** **True**  There is increased lactic acid production in this condition, which competes with uric acid for excretion by the renal tubule, leading to secondary hyperuricaemia which may even result in tophaceous deposits.

**D** **True**

E **False**   This is a characteristic feature of Type V disease (McArdle's disease), in which there is a skeletal myopathy.

**K14**  A **True**   This condition, which has been called 'male Turner syndrome', has many of the features of Turner syndrome (ovarian dysgenesis) including short stature, neck webbing, cubitus valgus, shield-shaped chest and widely spaced nipples. The karyotype is usually 46 XY or 46 XX. In the male the testes are often small and undescended, although fertility may be normal.

B **True**   A further shared feature with Turner syndrome.

C **False**   See (A).

D **True**   In this Noonan syndrome differs from Turner syndrome in which the commonest lesion is coarctation of the aorta.

E **False**

**K15**  A **False**   SSPE is not thought to be caused by mumps virus, but by measles. The condition may occur many years after an infection with measles, and there are very high levels of antibody to measles in the blood and cerebrospinal fluid. The condition is very rare and carries a poor prognosis.

B **True**   Herpes simplex causes a severe necrotizing encephalitis which frequently results in focal neurological signs such as a hemiplegia. The diagnosis should be suspected if the patient has a recent history of herpetic 'cold sores'. All cases of possible encephalitis should be treated as early as possible with acyclovir as this can improve the prognosis if encephalitis is due to herpes simplex.

C **False**   Measles encephalitis affects mainly the cerebrum. Varicella encephalitis has an especial predilection for the cerebellum, especially the vermis, and may present with truncal ataxia.

D **True**   Measles is said to cause encephalitis in about 1:1000 cases, and as this condition carries a significant mortality and morbidity it constitutes a strong argument for measles vaccination in developed countries. No such argument is necessary in developing countries where measles itself is a major cause of childhood mortality.

|   | E | True | Brain biopsy can confirm the diagnosis of herpes simplex encephalitis by demonstrating characteristic intranuclear inclusion bodies. However, treatment with acyclovir should already have been commenced, see (B) above, so brain biopsy is not essential for management. |

| K16 | A | False | In the majority of cases of Guillain–Barré syndrome there is total recovery of motor functions due to regeneration of lower motor neurons. Any degree of permanent paralysis is an exceptional event and probably occurs in less than 10% of cases. |
|   | B | False | Reflexes are decreased or absent as it is the lower motor neuron that is involved. |
|   | C | True | Paraesthesiae of hands and feet are a common feature of this syndrome, as is tenderness of the calf muscles. |
|   | D | True | Significant elevation of CSF protein without any cellular reaction is characteristic of this condition, although the first lumbar puncture may reveal normal protein levels. |
|   | E | True | This may lead to hypotension and tachycardia. |

| K17 | A | False | Tuberous sclerosis (epiloia, adenoma sebaceum) is inherited as an autosomal dominant, although a significant number of cases arise sporadically as mutations. The condition should be considered in all young children with epilepsy and mental retardation where there is no other obvious cause. Adenoma sebaceum may not be present in very young children, in which case the most important pointer to the condition is hypopigmented patches. Early diagnosis is important for the purpose of genetic counselling. |
|   | B | True | Galactosaemia is inherited as an autosomal recessive, and is a relatively rare condition with an incidence variously estimated at between 1:20 000 and 1:70 000. It presents in the first week of life with vomiting, lethargy and then jaundice, followed (if untreated) by liver failure and death. Delayed treatment may lead to survivors with mental retardation, cataracts and cirrhosis. All unwell jaundiced neonates should have their urine tested for reducing substances as a means of preventing these tragedies. |

C **False** Duchenne muscular dystrophy is inherited as an X-linked recessive, but mutations are relatively frequent, being responsible for the 30% of sporadic cases. The condition occurs in one in every 3000 males. Full family studies should be performed to try to find female carriers of the condition and to give genetic counselling.

D **True** Cystic fibrosis is the commonest serious condition inherited as an autosomal recessive in Caucasian populations. It occurs in 1:2000 births and the carrier rate in the population is 1:25. Pilot studies of neonatal screening programmes have been performed. The main benefit of such schemes is likely to be improved genetic counselling, although there is some evidence that earlier treatment carries long-term benefit.

E **False** Chronic granulomatous disease of childhood is a rare condition which is probably inherited mainly as a sex-linked recessive. The main defect in this condition is an inability of the child's polymorphs to kill pathogenic organisms after having ingested them, and this leads to chronic granulomata developing in lymph nodes.

K18 A **False** The sex incidence is 5:1 in favour of boys.

B **False** This is not an inflammatory condition, consisting as it does of avascular necrosis of portions of the femoral head.

C **True** It may also cause wasting of the quadriceps.

D **False** Straight X-rays may fail to demonstrate early Perthes' disease, whereas X-rays taken in the 'frog' position may succeed.

E **False** Perthes' disease usually occurs over the 4–8-year age range.

K19 A **False** The maximum number of brain cells is attained by 30 weeks of gestation, and all subsequent changes consist of increased differentiation, myelination and glial proliferation.

B **True** This is a reflection of the fact that the brain cells are so undifferentiated at the time of birth.

C **False** The head circumference increases very rapidly over the first 6 months then gradually slows down over the next 18 months.

D **True**

**E** **True** Convulsions should always be considered as a cause of apparent apnoeic attacks in the early neonatal period, especially when there is no obvious cause for the latter.

**K20** **A** **True** Addison's disease presents with hyperkalaemia and hyponatraemia, and hydrocortisone therapy leads to potassium loss and sodium retention.

**B** **False** Like all cells, red cells are rich in potassium and any acute haemolysis (as in transfusion reactions, haemolytic uraemic syndrome, etc.) can lead to dangerous degrees of hyperkalaemia.

**C** **True** Theophyllines, prednisolone and hydrocortisone and systemic $\beta_2$ agonists can all lead to hypokalaemia. Thus a patient with severe asthma on maintenance theophylline is at risk of hypokalaemia if, in an acute attack, systemic steroids and further theophylline are given.

**D** **False** In metabolic acidosis (e.g. untreated diabetic ketoacidosis) hydrogen ions cross into cells in exchange for potassium ions. This causes hyperkalaemia, which in DKA masks the fact that there is an underlying depletion of total body potassium.

**E** **True** This rare condition presents with failure to thrive, polyuria, polydipsia and constipation. The metabolic picture closely resembles primary hyperaldosteronism but unlike the latter condition there is no hypertension. There is profound hypokalaemia with hypochloraemic alkalosis.

# PAPER L
## QUESTIONS

**L1** Recognized causes of stridor include:
A a foreign body in the left main bronchus.
B *Haemophilus influenzae* infection.
C vascular ring.
D hypercalcaemia.
E *Corynebacterium diphtheriae* infection.

**L2** The following conditions are recognized causes of clubbing:
A untreated coeliac disease.
B asthma.
C fibrosing alveolitis.
D pyogenic lung abscess.
E biliary cirrhosis.

**L3** The following are recognized complications of infectious mononucleosis:
A splenic rupture during convalescence.
B encephalitis.
C respiratory obstruction.
D thrombocytopenia.
E erythematous rash if exposed to flucloxacillin.

**L4** Whooping cough (pertussis):
A may occur in the first month of life.
B has a mortality which is maximal between the ages of 1 and 3 years.
C should only be diagnosed if it is proved bacteriologically.
D should not be diagnosed in the absence of the characteristic whoop.
E characteristically is associated with a polymorphonuclear leukocytosis.

**L5** Cerebral abscess in childhood:
A may be secondary to congenital heart disease in which there is left-to-right shunting.
B should be treated with intrathecal amoxycillin.
C may result from frontal sinusitis.
D may benefit from treatment with metronidazole.
E should never be treated with chloramphenicol.

**L6**    A light-for-dates full-term baby is at particular risk from the following conditions:

A    hyaline membrane disease.
B    physiological jaundice.
C    milk aspiration.
D    hypoglycaemia.
E    apnoeic attacks.

**L7**    Recurrent apnoea of prematurity:

A    characteristically develops within the first 24 hours of life.
B    is more likely to occur in infants of less than 32 weeks' gestation.
C    usually responds to naloxone.
D    should be treated with 100% oxygen during attacks.
E    may be accentuated by the presence of a nasogastric tube.

**L8**    In tetralogy of Fallot:

A    there is usually a pansystolic murmur at the left sternal edge.
B    affected infants are usually cyanosed at birth.
C    cyanotic spells may be helped by propranolol.
D    both ventricles are usually hypertrophied.
E    chest X-ray characteristically shows pulmonary plethora.

**L9**    The following statements concerning ulcerative colitis in childhood are correct:

A    the small bowel is affected in about 15% of cases.
B    acute toxic dilatation of the colon is best managed medically.
C    erythema nodosum is a recognized feature.
D    prednisone by enema is an effective treatment.
E    if surgery is planned, attempts should be made to preserve as much of the colon as possible.

**L10**    The following conditions may cause a delayed bone age:

A    congenital adrenal hyperplasia.
B    hypothyroidism.
C    limb girdle muscular dystrophy.
D    psychosocial dwarfism.
E    craniopharyngioma.

**L11**    Regarding anaemia in childhood:

A    a haemoglobin concentration of 11 g/100 ml at the age of 3 months merits investigation.
B    iron supplements should be given to all breastfed infants for the first 6 months of life.
C    serum iron is characteristically raised and iron-binding capacity reduced in chronic haemolytic anaemias.
D    the majority of cases of iron deficiency anaemia in the first 2 years of childhood are nutritional in origin.

**E** in the treatment of iron deficiency anaemia, parenteral iron therapy raises the haemoglobin faster than oral iron.

**L12** The following statements concerning minimal change nephrotic syndrome are correct:
**A** macroscopic haematuria is a characteristic finding.
**B** hyaline casts are a recognized finding.
**C** the majority of patients will require treatment with cyclophosphamide.
**D** a mild degree of hypertension is characteristic.
**E** hypovolaemic shock can occur in the presence of peripheral oedema.

**L13** The following conditions can cause tetany:
**A** acute pancreatitis.
**B** bony metastases.
**C** chronic renal failure.
**D** hyperventilation.
**E** hyperparathyroidism.

**L14** The following isolated findings are to be regarded as abnormal:
**A** a non-retractile prepuce at 18 months.
**B** a patent anterior fontanelle at 12 months.
**C** an 8-week-old infant who has not smiled responsively.
**D** a child of 18 months who can only speak six words.
**E** an 8-month-old with no teeth.

**L15** In Down syndrome:
**A** the commonest congenital heart defect is patent ductus arteriosus.
**B** there is an increased incidence of acute lymphatic leukaemia.
**C** cases due to translocation are associated with increased maternal age.
**D** fetal blood sampling should be offered to all pregnant women over the age of 36 years.
**E** borderline clinical features suggest mosaicism.

**L16** The following are recognized complications of ventriculoatrial (VA) shunts for the treatment of hydrocephalus:
**A** meningitis.
**B** superior vena caval thrombosis.
**C** secondary polycythaemia.
**D** pulmonary hypertension.
**E** intraventricular haemorrhage.

**L17** The following are features of the Stevens–Johnson syndrome (erythema multiforme bullosum):
**A** purpura.
**B** urethritis.

**C** nephritis.
**D** conjunctivitis.
**E** association with primary atypical pneumonia.

**L18** **The following statements are true concerning antituberculous drug treatment:**
  **A** ethambutol may cause optic neuritis.
  **B** rifampicin may cause red urine.
  **C** rifampicin may cause hepatitis.
  **D** avian mycobacteria are usually sensitive to isoniazid.
  **E** the advent of newer drugs has led to isoniazid becoming a second-line drug in the UK at the present time.

**L19** **Regarding maternal-infant bonding:**
  **A** the first hour of life is a critical period for the infant to become attached to the mother.
  **B** admission to special care nurseries has been associated with an increased incidence of child abuse.
  **C** an infant aged 6 months should by this stage have developed an attachment to his mother of maximum intensity.
  **D** if a boy of 10 years is admitted to hospital his mother should be discouraged from staying in with him, to teach him to stand on his own feet.
  **E** if a child of 18 months can come into hospital on his own without showing undue distress this is evidence of excellent parenting prior to this event.

**L20** **The following are recognized complications of heat stroke in young children:**
  **A** peripheral circulatory failure.
  **B** pulmonary fibrosis.
  **C** disseminated intravascular coagulation.
  **D** brain damage.
  **E** metabolic alkalosis.

# PAPER L
## ANSWERS

**L1**  **A**  **False**   Stridor is caused by upper respiratory obstruction and consists of an inspiratory sound with a crowing or croaking quality. The commonest cause in paediatric practice is viral laryngitis or 'croup', which is most commonly due to parainfluenza type III virus infection. A foreign body in the left main bronchus will not cause stridor but may cause an audible wheeze. A foreign body impacted just above or below the larynx might very well cause stridor.

    **B**  **True**   In acute stridor in hospital paediatric practice, over 90% of cases will be viral and usually require supportive treatment only. However, roughly 5% of cases will be due to epiglottitis, a severe infection caused by *Haemophilus influenzae*, in which inflammation of the epiglottis and surrounding tissues is accompanied by septicaemia. Death from respiratory obstruction may be very rapid, at worst within 4 hours of the first symptom. Clinical features suggestive of the condition are disproportionate toxicity and reluctance to swallow with drooling of saliva.

    **C**  **True**   A rare cause of increasing stridor in the first 6 months of life is a congenital vascular ring which progressively compresses both the trachea and oesophagus. Barium swallow examination will reveal indentation of the column of barium. Definitive diagnosis requires angiocardiography and treatment is surgical.

    **D**  **False**   Hypercalcaemia does not cause stridor. Hypocalcaemia does, as a component part of tetany. Causes of hypocalcaemia in childhood include cow's milk tetany in the neonatal period, hypoparathyroidism and chronic renal failure.

E    **True**    Although virtually eliminated from the UK by immunization programmes, very occasional sporadic cases of diphtheria still occur. The commonest clinical presentation is with pharyngeal membrane, toxaemia and cervical adenopathy giving a 'bullneck' appearance. In addition the exotoxin produced causes myocarditis and a predominantly motor peripheral neuropathy. If the pharyngeal membrane extends to involve the larynx this may cause life-threatening respiratory obstruction.

L2    A    **True**    Treatment with a gluten-free diet usually leads to regression of clubbing.

B    **False**

C    **True**    While exceedingly rare, this condition has been reported in children.

D    **True**    Any suppurative lung condition can cause clubbing (other examples being empyema and bronchiectasis). Treatment of the underlying condition can lead to reversal of the clubbing.

E    **True**    Causes of biliary cirrhosis in childhood include biliary atresia and cystic fibrosis.

L3    A    **True**    Infectious mononucleosis commonly causes considerable enlargement of the spleen and any enlarged spleen is more likely to rupture than a normal spleen.

B    **True**    A subclinical encephalitis may contribute to the lethargy and depression in the convalescent period for which this disease is famous.

C    **True**    In the anginose variety, grossly enlarged tonsils with cellulitis of the neck can lead to obstruction necessitating intubation or tracheostomy. Systemic steroid therapy is justified in cases where this complication is a threat, and can lead to a dramatic improvement.

D    **True**

E    **False**    The antibiotics which are especially likely to cause a rash are the closely related ampicillin and amoxycillin.

L4    A    **True**    There is no transmitted maternal immunity in this condition, so neonates are susceptible. The short incubation period of 7 days means that it can easily develop in the first month of life.

**B** **False** The mortality is greatest in the first year of life. The true figure for mortality in this condition is uncertain, but in the pre-vaccination era mortality figures of between 1:100 and 1:1000 were recorded.

**C** **False** Whooping cough is a clinical diagnosis and bacteriological confirmation is only found in about 40% of cases.

**D** **False** Infants under 6 months tend not to whoop, and diagnosis rests on the characteristic nature of the cough, which is staccato and comes in prolonged bouts without any pause for inspiration.

**E** **False** The blood picture is typically that of a marked lymphocytosis, which is sometimes severe enough to raise the possibility of leukaemia ('leukaemoid reaction').

**L5** **A** **False** Cerebral abscess may occur in congenital heart disease but only when the shunting is right-to-left. This is because the filtering effect of the pulmonary circulation is bypassed, so that for instance a staphylococcus which enters the systemic circulation from a boil can pass unimpeded from the right side of the heart to the left, and thence to the brain. Pyogenic lung abscess and bronchiectasis predispose to cerebral abscess for similar reasons. Another possible cerebral complication of cyanotic congenital heart disease is cerebral venous sinus thrombosis secondary to polycythaemia.

**B** **False** There are very few situations where intrathecal antibiotics are indicated, and cerebral abscess is not one of them. Intrathecal streptomycin is used in tuberculous meningitis and intrathecal gentamicin may be used in Gram-negative meningitis in neonates. Otherwise, both for cerebral abscess and pyogenic meningitis, the main task is to select the correct antibiotic combination and to give it in high enough dosage intravenously. Localization of the abscess by CT scanning and possible drainage may also be indicated, as may therapy aimed at reducing cerebral oedema.

**C** **True** Frontal sinusitis may lead to a cerebral abscess in the frontal lobe and should always be treated energetically if there is any suggestion of osteitis of the frontal bones. Patients with compound skull fractures should receive prophylactic antibiotics for the same reason. Other conditions predisposing to cerebral abscess include chronic suppurative otitis media and facial or orbital cellulitis.

**D   True**   Cerebral abscesses frequently contain anaerobic organisms, including *Bacteroides* species. Metronidazole is extremely effective against these organisms and crosses the blood–brain barrier in sufficient concentrations to be effective.

**E   False**   Chloramphenicol is a very useful drug in both cerebral abscess and pyogenic meningitis because of its broad spectrum and excellent ability to cross both the inflamed and non-inflamed blood–brain barrier. The extremely small risk of marrow aplasia is hardly a contraindication in such life-threatening conditions. A more common practical hazard is the 'grey baby' or 'grey toddler' syndrome, which is a dose-related toxic effect and is usually due to an error in mental arithmetic in calculating the dose!

**L6   A   False**   Hyaline membrane disease is virtually confined to preterm infants and infants of diabetic mothers.

**B   False**   Light-for-dates, full-term infants have mature liver enzymes and are therefore at no increased risk of physiological jaundice, whereas the converse holds in preterm infants.

**C   False**   There is no reason why a light-for-dates, full-term infant should be more likely to aspirate milk than any other full-term infant.

**D   True**   Hypoglycaemia constitutes the main hazard in light-for-dates infants, especially those in whom there has been intrauterine malnutrition in the latter stages of pregnancy. Such infants have limited glycogen and fat stores, and are lively and hungry. They have relatively large heads for their body weight and have wrinkled subcutaneous tissue from loss of fat. Management is early milk feeding and hourly monitoring of blood glucose.

**E   False**   Light-for-dates infants have no increased tendency to apnoeic attacks, which are a complication of prematurity.

**L7   A   False**   Recurrent apnoea of prematurity typically develops at about 5–6 days of age. Apnoeic attacks developing earlier should be regarded as more likely to be secondary to an organic problem, e.g. infection, hypoglycaemia, convulsions, etc.

**B   True**   Preterm infants over 32 weeks' gestation are rarely troubled by apnoeic attacks.

C **False** Naloxone does not have a significant effect on recurrent apnoea of prematurity. It is, of course, effective on apnoea secondary to respiratory depression by narcotic drugs.

D **False** There is no justification for the practice of using 100% oxygen to resuscitate preterm infants with recurrent apnoeic attacks. This practice is a very good recipe for retrolental fibroplasia and is probably the chief cause in current neonatal practice. The infant should be resuscitated with air, or an appropriate air–oxygen mixture, if there is lung disease and a need for enriched oxygen supply.

E **True**

**L8** A **False** A pansystolic murmur at the left sternal edge is characteristic of a ventricular septal defect (VSD), and VSD is one of the features of tetralogy of Fallot. However, in this condition the VSD does not usually give rise to a murmur because the usual high-velocity left-to-right flow is replaced by a less vigorous right-to-left flow. A systolic murmur is usually present in Fallot's tetralogy but is due to the pulmonary stenosis. The murmur is therefore *ejection* in type, not pansystolic.

B **False** Infants with Fallot's tetralogy are usually pink at birth but develop cyanosis over the next few weeks or months, especially when feeding or crying. This sequence of events is probably a reflection of gradually increasing infundibular pulmonary stenosis.

C **True** Cyanotic spells are probably due to infundibular spasm, and propranolol has been shown to be valuable in preventing cyanotic spells, presumably by lessening the tendency to infundibular spasm. Intravenous propranolol can also be used as emergency treatment for a severe cyanotic spell. Morphine is probably preferable, combined with oxygen.

D **False** Only the right ventricle (and right atrium) are hypertrophied in tetralogy of Fallot.

E **False** Pulmonary oligaemia is one of the cardinal features of tetralogy of Fallot, and this is proportional to the severity of the pulmonary stenosis.

**L9** A **False** Ulcerative colitis only affects the large bowel. Crohn's disease can affect both small and large bowel.

|  | **B** | **False** | This life-threatening emergency is an indication for urgent colectomy. |
|---|---|---|---|
|  | **C** | **True** | Ulcerative colitis and Crohn's disease produce almost identical peripheral manifestations including erythema nodosum, arthritis, aphthous ulceration, and clubbing. In addition ulcerative colitis causes pyoderma gangrenosa. |
|  | **D** | **False** | Prednisone (like cortisone) is an inactive steroid unsuitable for topical use. Both can be used systemically because they are rendered active by the addition of an hydroxyl group by the liver, thereby becoming prednisolone and hydrocortisone respectively. These latter drugs are the forms which should therefore be used for topical therapy. |
|  | **E** | **False** | This statement would be justifiable in the context of Crohn's disease with respect to either the small or large bowel. However, the increased incidence of carcinoma of the colon in ulcerative colitis leads to the preferred surgical management being total colectomy with ileostomy. Occasionally preservation of the rectum and ileorectal anastomosis may be justifiable. |
| **L10** | **A** | **False** | In congenital adrenal hyperplasia there is a build-up of androgenic steroids which causes an advanced bone age. |
|  | **B** | **True** | Hypothyroidism causes retardation of linear growth and a delayed bone age, both of which are reversed by treatment with thyroxine. |
|  | **C** | **False** | |
|  | **D** | **True** | Psychosocial dwarfism in its severe form can cause significant delay in bone age with virtual arrest of linear growth. The precise mechanism is not fully understood but some cases show reduction in growth hormone levels. Treatment with an emotionally warm environment and adequate nutrition leads to reversal of the above changes. |
|  | **E** | **True** | Craniopharyngioma can cause a delayed bone age both by causing growth hormone deficiency and by causing secondary hypothyroidism. |

**L11** **A** **False** Erythropoiesis virtually ceases at birth and there is a steady drop in haemoglobin concentration to levels as low as 10 g/100 ml at 3 months, at which time erythropoiesis is restimulated and the haemoglobin concentration starts to rise again.

**B** **False** See (A). Because erythropoiesis ceases for the first 3 months of life, iron from senescent red cells is available to build up the iron stores for the period from 3 to 6 months, so there is no great need for iron supplements for full-term infants. It is probably also worth questioning the automatic assumption that infants need to be saturated with iron in their first year of life, as there is some evidence that a state of mild iron deficiency protects against bacterial infections.

**C** **True** When red cells are lysed in chronic haemolytic anaemias their iron remains in the body. In addition there is increased iron absorption from the gut. The resultant increased serum iron and saturated iron-binding capacity may increase susceptibility to bacterial infections.

**D** **True** Other causes include coeliac disease and gastrointestinal blood loss, e.g. from peptic ulceration of a Meckel's diverticulum.

**E** **False** The limiting factor in the rate of rise of haemoglobin is the rate at which the bone marrow can utilize the iron given. There is therefore no difference in the rate of rise of haemoglobin with oral or parenteral iron and there are few indications for the latter in paediatric practice in view of its expense, unpleasantness (if given by intramuscular injection) and possible danger (if given as an intravenous infusion).

**L12** **A** **False** Macroscopic haematuria is extremely rare in minimal change nephrotic syndrome. Microscopic haematuria occurs in less than 20% of cases and is usually transient.

**B** **True**

**C** **False** The majority of children will respond to steroids and will eventually attain remission, possibly after one or two relapses. Cyclophosphamide is only considered in a minority of those children who are dependent on steroids and who are running into trouble with steroid toxicity.

**D   False**

**E   True**   In cases with marked hypoalbuminaemia and severe peripheral oedema, hypovolaemic circulatory failure can occur, and should be anticipated and prevented with salt-free albumin infusions. These should be covered with frusemide as there is a real risk of hypervolaemia with a too-rapid return of oedema fluid to the vascular compartment.

**L13   A   True**   The clinical syndrome of tetany can result from any condition in which there is a fall in the ionized calcium in the blood. This can occur in acute pancreatitis because fatty acids liberated from autolysed omental fat bind calcium ions causing hypocalcaemia.

**B   False**   Bony metastases cause hypercalcaemia and do not cause tetany.

**C   True**   In chronic renal failure there is retention of phosphate which leads to a reduction in both total plasma and ionized calcium, which can result in tetany. The usual concurrent metabolic acidosis will tend to work in the opposite direction by raising the ionized calcium. Any vomiting illness in a patient with chronic renal failure may precipitate tetany by causing a metabolic alkalosis.

**D   True**   Hyperventilation causes a drop in $P$aco$_2$ leading to a respiratory alkalosis. This can reduce the ionized calcium sufficiently to cause tetany, which is a common feature of the 'hyperventilation syndrome'. Treatment consists of persuading the patient to rebreathe from a paper bag, or else to calm down sufficiently to stop hyperventilating.

**E   False**   Hyperparathyroidism causes a raised plasma calcium and therefore does not cause tetany. Hypoparathyroidism does the opposite and so *can* cause tetany.

**L14   A   False**   The prepuce is adherent to the glans penis for the first year of life. A plane of cleavage develops spontaneously over the second and third years of life. Forcible attempts at retraction should be avoided, as should unnecessary circumcision.

**B   False**   The anterior fontanelle usually closes at about 18 months of age.

**C   True**   Smiling responsively is one of the most important early milestones and should occur within the first 6 weeks of life. It is a better prognostic indicator of future intellectual development than measures of gross motor development.

**D   False**   Speaking six words at 18 months is within the normal range of language development. Between 18 and 24 months many more individual words are usually acquired, together with the ability to link words in short sentences.

**E   False**   The average age of appearance of the first tooth is 6 months but there is a wide range of normality, from babies born with a tooth to normal infants with no teeth by their first birthday.

**L15   A   False**   Approximately 20% of cases of Down syndrome have associated congenital heart disease. The commonest varieties are ventricular septal defect, followed by atrial septal defect and Fallot's tetralogy.

**B   True**   There is a markedly increased incidence of acute lymphatic leukaemia in children with Down syndrome; the incidence is 10–18 times greater than in normal children, giving a risk of roughly 1 child in 2000 with Down syndrome contracting leukaemia.

**C   False**   95% of cases of Down syndrome are due to non-disjunction and this form of the syndrome is definitely associated with increased maternal age. Only about 3% are due to translocation, and this mechanism is *not* associated with increased maternal age. Most cases of Down syndrome occurring to mothers in their twenties are still due to non-disjunction.

**D   False**   Fetal blood sampling is a quite inappropriate procedure to suggest for the antenatal diagnosis of Down syndrome. Instead, amniocentesis is usually offered to mothers in their late thirties with a view to possible termination of affected offspring. It would probably not be appropriate to *perform* amniocentesis in a mother who would definitely refuse a termination because of the slight but defininite risk of accidentally inducing an abortion.

**E** **True** About 1% of cases of Down syndrome are mosaics, i.e. they possess different cell lines, some with normal chromosomes and some with trisomic cells. Mosaics can cover the whole spectrum of clinical and developmental variation between the two extremes of a clear case of Down syndrome and a normal child. They are probably responsible for most of the reports of children with Down syndrome with relatively high IQs.

**L16** **A** **True** The meningitis which complicates VA shunts may be difficult to eradicate. The range of organisms differs from the usual childhood meningitis, and often includes *Staphylococcus albus*, which characteristically causes a low-grade infection with splenomegaly. Management consists of removal of the infected valve, treatment of the meningitis and ventriculitis, and replacement with a new shunt.

**B** **True**

**C** **False**

**D** **True** Pulmonary hypertension occurs as a result of repeated small pulmonary emboli arising from the lower end of the shunt system. Such episodes should be detected early, the VA shunt removed, and replaced by a ventriculoperitoneal shunt.

**E** **True** Too rapid a decompression of severe hydrocephalus can lead to the complication of intraventricular haemorrhage which occurs as a result of the rapid fall in intraventricular pressure.

**L17** **A** **False** The rash in this condition is a vesicular or bullous eruption on an erythematous base, classically giving the so-called 'target lesions'. Purpura is not a feature of the Stevens–Johnson syndrome.

**B** **True** In this condition there is inflammation at mucocutaneous junctions, usually affecting the mouth, eyes and urethra. Urinary retention may be a problem.

**C** **False** Nephritis is not a feature of this condition.

**D   True**   Conjunctivitis is one of the main features of the Stevens–Johnson syndrome, and may lead to corneal involvement and possible blindness. It constitutes an indication for systemic steroid therapy which usually has a beneficial effect on the disease process.

**E   True**   Primary atypical pneumonia, often due to *Mycoplasma pneumoniae*, is one of the commonest clinical associations of the Stevens–Johnson syndrome. If it is present, it is reasonable to treat with erythromycin in case it is due to *Mycoplasma pneumoniae*.

**L18   A   True**   Although ethambutol is a very effective antituberculous drug, this complication is a definite disadvantage, and at present rifampicin and isoniazid are probably the first-choice combination in childhood.

**B   True**

**C   True**

**D   False**   These organisms usually cause cervical adenopathy. They are of low pathogenicity and they are usually highly resistant to all the usual antituberculous drugs. The treatment of choice is therefore surgical.

**E   False**   See (A). Isoniazid remains a definite drug of first choice for most situations.

**L19   A   False**   A distinction should be made between maternal-infant *bonding*, and infant-mother *attachment*. There is evidence that the first hour of life is a sensitive (but not totally critical) period for a mother to 'bond' to her infant, and that this process can occur optimally at this time. However, the human infant is far too undifferentiated to develop a significant attachment to anyone at this time. Significant attachment behaviour begins at around 6 months and grows in intensity to a peak at around 18 months. It will be seen that 'bonding' and 'attachment' are not synonymous, and proceed according to different time scales.

**B   True**   Early evidence for the importance of maternal-infant bonding came from these observations. Hopefully the more liberal regimes of present-day special care nurseries will reduce this association.

**C** **False** See (A).

**D** **False** It is difficult to think of any justification for this statement. Even if the mother has clearly been indulging in over-protective behaviour, this would be better tackled gently during her son's convalescent period rather than in the crisis situation occasioned by admission. If the admission is an emergency, e.g. diabetic ketosis, status asthmaticus, then it would be natural for a parent to wish to stay with the child, at least till the crisis is over. Any serious illness or crisis can lead to emotional regression (even in adults) and therefore the chronological age becomes less relevant.

**E** **False** On the contrary, such an observation throws serious doubt on the quality of the previous parenting, on both the strength of parent-child bonding and of child-parent attachment. A normal child who has experienced good parenting should be virtually inseparable from his parents at 18 months, and they from him.

**L20** **A** **True** Young infants who are well-wrapped or exposed to high environmental temperatures and who then develop a virus infection are at risk of this condition which may present as convulsions, shock or even as a 'cot death'. Under the age of 6 months, when the convulsive threshold of the brain is high, the presentation is more likely to be with shock, and above this age with convulsions which may be prolonged and difficult to control. Metabolic *acidosis* and raised hepatic enzymes are characteristic. Disseminated intravascular coagulation with renal failure leads to a high mortality in established forms of this condition. Survivors may have severe brain damage. Whether the very similar, recently described 'haemorrhagic shock – encephalopathy syndrome' is in fact a different clinical entity or simply a manifestation of hyperpyrexia remains a matter for debate.

**B** **False** See (A).

**C** **True** See (A).

**D** **True** See (A).

**E** **False** See (A).

# PAPER M
## QUESTIONS

**M1**  **In childhood gastroenteritis:**
    **A**  isolation of pathogenic *E. coli* is an indication for antibiotic treatment.
    **B**  drowsiness out of proportion to the degree of clinical dehydration suggests hypertonic dehydration.
    **C**  marked sunken eyes and diminished skin turgor suggest that dehydration is about 5%.
    **D**  glucose electrolyte solution is markedly superior to sucrose electrolyte solution in oral rehydration.
    **E**  children should be kept in hospital until the stools have returned to normal.

**M2**  **The differential diagnosis of a previously well 2-year-old child who has become moribund over 18 hours will include:**
    **A**  appendicitis.
    **B**  the nephrotic syndrome.
    **C**  meningococcal septicaemia.
    **D**  Henoch–Schönlein purpura.
    **E**  measles pneumonia.

**M3**  **The following statements are correct:**
    **A**  ileal stenosis is a recognized complication of accidental iron poisoning.
    **B**  chronic lead poisoning causes a punctate basophilia.
    **C**  poisoning with paracetamol characteristically results in cardiac arrhythmias.
    **D**  poisoning with diphenoxylate (Lomotil) characteristically causes fixed dilated pupils.
    **E**  ingestion of metoclopramide (Maxolon) may result in oculogyric crises.

**M4**  **Tuberculous meningitis in childhood:**
    **A**  usually occurs within 6 months of the primary infection.
    **B**  is associated with a negative Mantoux test in over 90% of cases.
    **C**  occurs in over 50% of cases of miliary tuberculosis.
    **D**  is associated with a normal CSF glucose.
    **E**  may benefit from systemic steroid therapy as an adjuvant to antituberculous drugs.

**M5**    **With regard to Wilms' tumour (nephroblastoma):**

A    there is a recognized association with aniridia.

B    repeated palpation of the tumour should be avoided.

C    the main drugs used in treatment are vinblastine and cytosine arabinoside.

D    the 5-year survival rate for children with Stage I tumours is about 30%.

E    the commonest presentation is with an abdominal mass.

**M6**    **In the management of hyaline membrane disease (HMD):**

A    tolazoline may lead to systemic hypertension.

B    early use of continuous positive airways pressure (CPAP) may reduce the need for subsequent ventilatory support.

C    antibiotics improve ventilation–perfusion ratios.

D    the illness may be expected to increase in severity for the first 5 days.

E    corticosteroids used postnatally have a beneficial effect on the course of the disease.

**M7**    **The following are recognized causes of the floppy infant syndrome:**

A    dystonia musculorum deformans.

B    maternal myasthenia gravis.

C    limb girdle muscular dystrophy.

D    maternal benzodiazepine therapy.

E    Werdnig–Hoffman disease.

**M8**    **In patent ductus arteriosus in neonates:**

A    in term infants, spontaneous closure is likely at any time in the first 12 months of life.

B    prostaglandins may be used to close the duct in preterm infants.

C    pulsus paradoxus is a characteristic finding.

D    a high arterial $Po_2$ may help the duct to close in early infancy.

E    surgery is indicated if pulmonary hypertension leads to reversal of shunting.

**M9**    **The following statements concerning respiratory tract infections in children are correct:**

A    acute epiglottitis is caused by *Haemophilus influenzae*.

B    the commonest cause of acute viral laryngitis ('croup') is the parainfluenza virus.

C    infections with *Mycoplasma pneumoniae* respond to treatment with amoxycillin.

D    acute bronchiolitis is unusual over the age of 2 years.

E    measles characteristically causes a lobar pneumonia.

**M10**    **Hurler syndrome (gargoylism) may be characterized by:**

A    recurrent hypoglycaemia.

B    deafness.

**C** clouding of the cornea.
**D** macroglossia.
**E** beak-shaped deformities of vertebrae.

**M11 In acute appendicitis in childhood:**
**A** the characteristic presentation is with colicky abdominal pain in the right iliac fossa.
**B** vomiting typically precedes the onset of pain.
**C** rectal examination is mandatory in every patient who is to be subjected to surgery.
**D** pyuria is a recognized finding in children with a pelvic abscess.
**E** the obturator test is designed to detect the presence of an inflamed retrocaecal appendix.

**M12 Bone age:**
**A** is more advanced in girls than in boys of the same age.
**B** is characteristically retarded in girls with untreated congenital adrenal hyperplasia.
**C** is a better predictor of final adult height than height-for-age.
**D** may be retarded by emotional deprivation.
**E** may be retarded in chronic renal failure.

**M13 Nephroblastoma (Wilms' tumour):**
**A** may be suspected by finding raised levels of urinary catecholamines.
**B** may be associated with aniridia.
**C** occurs most commonly in the age range 5–10 years.
**D** may embolize to the lungs.
**E** may show calcification on straight abdominal X-ray.

**M14 In juvenile chronic polyarthritis:**
**A** a common presentation is with recurrent erythematous rashes coupled with pyrexia.
**B** the distal interphalangeal joints are classically involved.
**C** in the acute stage, joint involvement is typically 'flitting'.
**D** rheumatoid factor is negative in over 80% of cases.
**E** the disease tends to improve in the early teens.

**M15 Galactosaemia:**
**A** is inherited as an autosomal dominant.
**B** can be excluded by a negative Clinistix test on urine.
**C** is a recognized cause of cataract.
**D** may lead to cardiomyopathy.
**E** may lead to mental retardation.

**M16 Regarding the surface markings of the chest contents:**
**A** the trachea bifurcates at the level of the fourth costal cartilages.

B   the oblique fissure starts posteriorly at the level of the
    spine of T4.
C   the horizontal fissure on the right is level with the junction
    of the sternum with the third costal cartilage.
D   the liver edge is easily palpable in 2-year-olds.
E   crepitations heard posteriorly at the level of T3 signify
    pathology in the upper lobe.

**M17   The following observations should be regarded as abnormal:**
A   temper tantrums in a 2-year-old.
B   feeding negativism in a 7-year-old.
C   asking repeated questions about life and death in a 4-year-
    old.
D   sadness lasting several weeks in a 9-year-old.
E   bedwetting in a 7-year-old.

**M18   Osteogenesis imperfecta Type I:**
A   is typically inherited as a Mendelian recessive trait.
B   is a recognized cause of deafness.
C   is characteristically associated with blue irises.
D   is characterized by fractures that heal at the normal rate.
E   is associated with hydrocephalus.

**M19   In petit mal epilepsy:**
A   attacks are often regarded as simple 'day-dreaming' by
    teachers.
B   retrograde amnesia is characteristic.
C   attacks may be precipitated by over-breathing.
D   the drug of first choice is carbamazepine.
E   attacks virtually never persist into adulthood.

**M20   In the child with cerebral palsy:**
A   spastic diplegia has a worse prognosis for intellectual
    development than other types.
B   in cases of congenital hemiplegia spasticity is likely to be
    maximal by the age of 3 months.
C   measles vaccine is contraindicated.
D   pseudobulbar palsy is likely in cases of congenital
    hemiplegia.
E   sensory loss of 'cortical' type may occur in children with
    spastic hemiplegia.

# PAPER M
## ANSWERS

**M1**  **A**  **False**  There are very few indications for antibiotic therapy in gastroenteritis as most studies show that such therapy fails to affect the clinical course and may even prolong the carrier state.

  **B**  **True**  The signs of 'clinical dehydration' are really those of extracellular fluid depletion, and are best seen in isotonic dehydration. In hypertonic dehydration the extracellular fluid volume is preserved until late because of movement of water out of the cells. Accordingly the *water* depletion that has occurred is difficult to detect clinically, and undue drowsiness in a child who appears only slightly dehydrated is an important pointer to possible hypertonic dehydration.

  **C**  **False**  These signs indicate dehydration of at least 10%; 5% dehydration is barely clinically detectable.

  **D**  **False**  For practical purposes, sucrose-based fluids are as effective as those made with glucose, as the number of children who have transient inability to digest sucrose is very small indeed. This is fortunate as it means health education aimed at preventing and treating dehydration can encourage the use of home-based recipes using sucrose. This is of tremendous importance for developing countries, and is not without importance in developed countries.

  **E**  **False**  The main reasons for a child to be in hospital with gastroenteritis are: (1) because he/she needs intravenous fluids; (2) because he/she has a severe attack and needs observation in case of sudden deterioration; and (3) for social reasons, e.g. parental anxiety or incompetence. There is no need to keep a child in hospital if none of these conditions is operative, and to keep a child till the stool is normal is quite unnecessary.

**M2**   **A**   **True**   Acute appendicitis does occur at this age and is usually not diagnosed initially, often being regarded as gastroenteritis. Perforation with peritonitis leading to peripheral circulatory failure can occur rapidly, certainly within 18 hours of the first symptom.

    **B**   **False**   While known cases of nephrotic syndrome can deteriorate rapidly after having been significantly hypoproteinaemic for some time, such cases will always have been previously symptomatic. It is virtually impossible for the nephrotic syndrome to cause such rapid deterioration 'de novo'.

    **C**   **True**   Meningococcal septicaemia is quite capable of causing death from peripheral circulatory failure within less than 18 hours of the first symptom. It is a fulminating condition frequently complicated by disseminated intravascular coagulation (DIC).

    **D**   **False**   Henoch–Schönlein purpura is an extremely unlikely cause of such a rapid deterioration. However, once the condition is established, gastrointestinal bleeding with shock is a possibility.

    **E**   **False**   Children with measles usually have a prodromal illness lasting 3–4 days before the rash appears, and the most dangerous complication of bacterial bronchopneumonia would be unlikely to occur before the 5th or 6th day of the illness.

**M3**   **A**   **True**   Iron salts cause acute necrosis of the portions of the alimentary tract with which they come in contact, and late sequelae include fibrotic scarring and stenosis of the small intestine.

    **B**   **True**   Lead interferes with haemoglobin synthesis causing a hypochromic anaemia with a mild haemolytic picture. The latter results in reticulocytosis and basophilic stippling of red cells.

    **C**   **False**   Paracetamol causes hepatic necrosis. The most likely drugs to cause cardiac arrhythmias when ingested by children are tricyclic antidepressants, either prescribed for parents for depression, or for older siblings for enuresis.

    **D**   **False**   Diphenoxylate is one of the opiates and is used (somewhat unnecessarily) as a symptomatic treatment for diarrhoea. It causes pinpoint pupils and respiratory depression in overdose. Its effects are reversed by naloxone.

E **True** Oculogyric crises are often wrongly diagnosed as hysteria. They may also follow therapy with drugs of the phenothiazine group.

M4 A **True**

B **False** The Mantoux reaction is usually strongly positive, and is only likely to be diminished or negative in the patient who is extremely ill and cachectic due to late diagnosis.

C **True** For this reason all cases of miliary tuberculosis should have their CSF examined, even if meningitis is not clinically apparent.

D **False** The CSF glucose is characteristically decreased, which differentiates this condition from viral meningitis.

E **True** It is reasonably orthodox to use systemic steroid therapy in the hope of decreasing the meningeal reaction and the chance of adhesions, cranial nerve palsies and the risk of spinal block.

M5 A **True** Wilms' tumour is also associated with hemihypertrophy and Beckwith syndrome.

B **True** Repeated palpation is thought to increase the chance of haematogenous metastases to the lungs.

C **False** Vincristine is the drug used at the time of surgery, and actinomycin, adriamycin and cyclophosphamide are used in the presence of metastases. Radiotherapy is also used.

D **False** Stage I disease (i.e. cases in which disease is limited to the kidney) has a 5-year survival rate of 80–90%.

E **True** Most cases are symptomatic until a mass is felt on routine examination. Otherwise, cases may present with fever, anorexia, weight loss or haematuria.

M6 A **False** Tolazoline is a pulmonary vasodilator and its chief side effect and disadvantage is systemic *hypotension*. It may be useful in cases of severe HMD receiving maximal ventilatory support, as it can reverse reactive pulmonary vasoconstriction, improve lung perfusion and thereby improve the blood gases.

B **True** It is generally agreed that the early use of CPAP in HMD has a beneficial effect and can provide the main form of support for infants who would otherwise have needed artificial ventilation.

    **C**  **False**   Some centres use antibiotics routinely in all cases of HMD and others do not. The rationale for the use of antibiotics is (1) prophylactic and (2) because it is difficult to be certain that in an individual case the respiratory distress is not due to infection such as Group B streptococcal pneumonia. There is no evidence that antibiotics have any beneficial effect on pure hyaline membrane disease.

    **D**  **False**   The severity of HMD usually reaches a peak at 24–48 hours, remains static for a further 24 hours and then gradually begins to wane, as the beneficial effects of resynthesis of surfactant become apparent.

    **E**  **False**   There is no evidence that corticosteroid therapy is effective in established HMD. However, there is evidence that steroids administered to the mother before delivery can reduce the incidence and severity of HMD in preterm infants. Steroids can also be effective in bronchopulmonary dysplasia but this is a different issue, even though it is a common *complication* of HMD.

**M7**  **A**  **False**   Dystonia musculorum deformans is a rare extrapyramidal disorder which presents in early childhood with abnormal posture of one or other limb, affecting the legs more commonly than the arms. There is a familial tendency. The condition is so rare and bizarre that it is commonly regarded as hysteria or malingering for months or years before the correct diagnosis is made. This condition does not cause any abnormalities of tone in early infancy.

    **B**  **True**   A significant number of infants born to mothers with myasthenia gravis will themselves develop a transient myasthenia-like illness lasting for up to 6 weeks. This situation is thus a cause of the floppy infant syndrome. At-risk infants should be observed closely for feeding and respiratory difficulties and if symptoms develop then a test dose of edrophonium (Tensilon) should be given.

    **C**  **False**   Limb girdle muscular dystrophy does not affect infants or young children, usually presenting after the age of 10 with weakness and wasting of the pelvic and shoulder girdles. This condition is inherited as an autosomal recessive.

**D   True**   Benzodiazepines have been shown to cross the placenta and to be capable of affecting the infant quite severely. Given to mothers in high doses, diazepam has been associated with respiratory depression severe enough to require ventilatory support. As diazepam is a muscle relaxant it can cause floppiness in neonates. It also causes poor sucking and reduced thermogenesis in response to cold. It is probable that low-dose long-term use in pregnancy can also cause these features. Nitrazepam (Mogadon) used for antenatal night sedation has also been reported to have these effects.

**E   True**   Werdnig–Hoffman disease (Type I spinal muscular atrophy) is a classic cause of the floppy infant syndrome. It is inherited as an autosomal recessive. Mothers of affected infants frequently report diminished fetal movements. At birth the infant is hypotonic and tends to slip through the hands. Fasciculation of tongue muscles is characteristic. The prognosis is very poor, with death from bronchopneumonia likely by the second year of life.

**M8   A   False**   In term infants spontaneous closure of a patent duct may occur in the first few days of life, but is thereafter increasingly unlikely to occur. In preterm infants, spontaneous closure may occur over the first 3 months of life.

**B   False**   Prostaglandins keep the duct open and are used therapeutically in cases of congenital heart disease where a patent duct is vital to survival pending surgery, e.g. severe preductal coarctation. Indomethacin, which is a prostaglandin synthetase inhibitor, is used for pharmacological closure of ducts in preterm infants. It is most likely to be effective in infants between 30 and 35 weeks' gestation who are less than 3 weeks old.

**C   False**   The pulse in patent ductus arteriosus is characteristically large volume and bounding. Pulsus paradoxus is not a feature. Pulsus paradoxus occurs in cardiac tamponade or conditions like severe asthma where there is diminution of venous return to the heart made worse by inspiration.

**D   True**   A high arterial $P_{O_2}$ is the usual physiological stimulus to duct closure in normal infants. Persistent hypoxia (as in severe cases of the respiratory distress syndrome) and prematurity may combine to prevent this normal physiological process from occurring.

**E** **False** Early signs of pulmonary hypertension are an urgent indication for investigation and possible surgery. However, it is too late for surgery once the right-sided pressure exceeds that on the left and reversal of shunting has occurred (Eisenmenger syndrome). If the duct were to be closed surgically in such infants they would develop right-sided heart failure which would carry a poor prognosis. If the duct were left open, such children would survive into adulthood with differential cyanosis from a right-to-left shunt through the duct.

**M9** **A** **True** This condition is capable of causing rapid deterioration and death within a few hours of onset. Features which help to distinguish it from the far commoner viral croup are: (1) the child looks more ill, (2) difficulty swallowing with drooling of saliva, (3) rapid deterioration, (4) less likely to be preceded by a viral upper respiratory tract infection. Although Hib vaccine is reducing the incidence of this condition in the UK, it can be expected still to occur in non-immune older children. It has even been described in adults. *Haemophilus influenzae* can usually be isolated from throat swabs and also from blood cultures as there is usually a coexisting septicaemia.

**B** **True** Parainfluenza virus Type III is the commonest cause of viral croup although numerous other viruses are occasionally responsible.

**C** **False** *Mycoplasma pneumoniae* infections are common in childhood and can cause otitis media, bronchiolitis, tonsillitis, pyrexia of unknown origin and primary atypical pneumonia. The latter condition is characterized by a very irritant dry cough, dry crepitations over the lower zones posteriorly and patchy shadowing in the lower zones on X-ray. Erythromycin is the drug of choice. The only other antibiotic effective in this condition is tetracycline which is relatively contraindicated in childhood.

**D** **True** Acute bronchiolitis occurs mainly in the first year of life with a smaller number of cases occurring in the second year. It is very unusual for it to occur after the second birthday. It may affect the same child twice, but in an apparent third attack consideration should be given to regarding the case as one of asthma.

**E  False**  The main cause of lobar pneumonia is the pneumococcus. Measles can affect the lower respiratory tract in several ways. It frequently causes a laryngotracheobronchitis. It may cause a true viral (giant cell) pneumonia; this condition is rare in healthy children but more likely in immunosuppressed children. Far more commonly, measles leads to a secondary bacterial bronchopneumonia.

**M10  A  False**  Hurler syndrome causes coarse facies, severe mental retardation and dwarfism. Although hepatomegaly and splenomegaly are constant features, there is no significant problem with hypoglycaemia.

**B  True**  This condition is inherited as an autosomal recessive and clouding of the cornea is a characteristic feature. Hunter syndrome (mucopolysaccharidosis Type II) is by contrast inherited as an X-linked recessive and does not have corneal clouding.

**C  True**  See (B).

**D  True**  This increases the impression of mental retardation because the tongue tends to protrude.

**E  True**  These are apparent on lateral X-ray of the spine, and frequently result in an angular kyphosis.

While the basic condition is usually regarded as untreatable, a few cases appear to have had their metabolic defect cured by marrow transplantation.

**M11  A  False**  Pain due to appendicular colic is referred to the midline at the level of the umbilicus. When pain is eventually felt in the right iliac fossa it is of a constant nature and is secondary to irritation of the parietal peritoneum in that region.

**B  False**  Vomiting is a late feature of acute appendicitis, but may be an early feature in mesenteric adenitis.

**C  False**  Rectal examination is mainly intended to reveal a pelvic appendicitis in someone with no abdominal tenderness. It does not add useful information in the majority of classic cases in whom surgery is already planned.

**D  True**  A pelvic abscess pressing on the bladder or lower ureter can result in sterile pyuria.

**E  False**  The obturator test is meant to reveal pelvic peritonitis. The test for the retrocaecal appendix is the psoas test.

**M12**  **A**  **True**    This parallels the fact that puberty generally occurs slightly earlier in girls than in boys.

  **B**  **False**    In this situation there will be excessive secretion of anabolic steroids by the adrenal cortex, leading to advanced bone age.

  **C**  **True**    An isolated height-for-age reading is a poor predictor of adult height. Bone age allows an estimate to be made of the likely age of puberty and thus gives additional evidence on which to predict adult height.

  **D**  **True**    Emotional deprivation may stunt linear growth, and bone age will be correspondingly retarded. These effects are most marked between 1 and 4 years of age when a child's emotional needs are maximal. Rapid catch-up of linear growth is possible.

  **E**  **True**    Any severe systemic illness may retard bone age.

**M13**  **A**  **False**    Urinary catecholamines may be raised in neuroblastoma, which usually arises from the adrenal medulla, but are normal in nephroblastoma, which consists of embryonic renal tissue. The latter may secrete renin and cause hypertension.

  **B**  **True**    There is a definite association between aniridia and nephroblastoma.

  **C**  **False**    60% of cases of nephroblastoma present before the age of 3 years.

  **D**  **True**    Nephroblastoma characteristically invades the renal vein and may cause pulmonary emboli of both blood clots and tumour tissue. Repeated palpation is contraindicated as it increases the chance of embolization.

  **E**  **True**    Calcification on straight abdominal X-ray may occur in up to 15% of cases of nephroblastoma.

**M14**  **A**  **True**    Juvenile chronic polyarthritis may initially present with recurrent rashes and fever with or without joint involvement. Diagnostic confusion may be caused by *Mycoplasma pneumoniae* infection which can produce a similar clinical picture, including arthritis.

  **B**  **False**    As with adult forms of the disease, distal interphalangeal joints are characteristically spared.

    **C**   **False**   A 'flitting' polyarthritis is typical of acute rheumatic fever, i.e. inflammation leaves one joint and moves on to another. In rheumatoid arthritis the joint involvement is typically cumulative.

    **D**   **True**   The diagnosis of this condition is essentially clinical.

    **E**   **True**

**M15**   **A**   **False**   Galactosaemia is inherited as an autosomal recessive.

    **B**   **False**   The Clinistix test is specific for glucose and is therefore of no help in diagnosing galactosaemia. Use of a Clinitest tablet will be helpful as it is a non-specific test for reducing substances, and galactose being a reducing sugar will give a positive result.

    **C**   **True**   Cataract is an extremely likely complication of untreated galactosaemia.

    **D**   **False**   Cardiomyopathy occurs in some forms of glycogen storage disease but is not a recognized feature of galactosaemia.

    **E**   **True**   Early diagnosis and treatment with a galactose-free diet should prevent this complication.

**M16**   **A**   **False**   The trachea bifurcates at the level of the second costal cartilage and its junction with the manubriosternal joint.

    **B**   **False**   It starts at the level of the spine of T2.

    **C**   **False**   The horizontal fissure is level with the fourth costal cartilage.

    **D**   **True**   At this age the liver is $2\frac{1}{2}$ times its adult size relative to the rest of the body.

    **E**   **False**   Physical signs in this area will reflect pathology in the apical segment of the lower lobe.

**M17**   **A**   **False**   Temper tantrums are virtually normal at this age.

    **B**   **True**   Feeding negativism is normal in toddlerhood but abnormal thereafter. It usually signifies parental inability to tolerate their child's choice of this battleground upon which to assert his need for autonomy. If it has persisted till the age of 7 it could last throughout childhood unless there is intervention.

| | C | **False** | This is entirely normal at this age, which is a time of great curiosity on such matters, as well as on more mundane matters. Questioning about life and death in, e.g. a 9-year-old child, would be more abnormal. |
|---|---|---|---|
| | D | **True** | A 9-year-old is in the middle of the so-called 'latency' period in which life should be relatively simple and happy. Persisting sadness should therefore be taken seriously, as it probably should be at any age. |
| | E | **True** | While 10% of 5-year-olds and 5% of 9-year-olds wet the bed, this does not mean that it is normal. It is best to regard most children as capable of achieving nocturnal bladder control by the age of 4, and to wish to help those children who have not as early as possible. Certainly avoidable emotional problems should be sought and dealt with if possible. |
| **M18** | A | **False** | Type I is caused by an autosomal dominant gene occurring as a sporadic mutation. |
| | B | **True** | Deafness is a common feature in middle age due to otosclerosis. |
| | C | **False** | The irises are normal in colour. The sclerae are pale blue instead of white due to abnormally thin collagen. |
| | D | **True** | Although the bones fracture easily, callus formation and healing of the fractures occurs normally. |
| | E | **False** | Although the head may appear large at birth with temporal bossing, there is no association with hydrocephalus. |
| **M19** | A | **True** | Teachers are ideally placed to diagnose this condition but because it is often so minor in nature it is very easy for them to dismiss attacks as innocent. Frequent attacks can obviously impede educational progress. |
| | B | **False** | There is no retrograde amnesia, just amnesia for events occurring during the attack. |
| | C | **True** | Over-breathing is a useful manoeuvre to provoke attacks, e.g. in a clinic setting. |
| | D | **False** | Carbamazepine is not effective in this condition although it is a very useful drug for grand mal and temporal lobe epilepsy. Ethosuximide remains one of the drugs of choice in petit mal epilepsy and is said to be effective in 90% of cases. Sodium valproate is also effective in petit mal. |

**E**  **False**  Although many children grow out of petit mal epilepsy, in an appreciable number attacks persist into adult life.

**M20**  **A**  **False**  In general, spastic tetraplegia has the worst prognosis for intellectual development; this is understandable as of necessity a great area of brain tissue must have been involved to produce the motor deficit.

    **B**  **False**  The affected limb is likely to be flaccid for the first 2–3 months of life and spasticity only begins to develop from 3 months onwards, becoming maximal at around the age of 12 months.

    **C**  **False**  Pre-existing cerebral palsy is not a contraindication to measles vaccine.

    **D**  **False**  Pseudobulbar palsy is a condition in which there are bilateral upper motor neuron lesions of the lower cranial nerves, and thus does not occur in hemiplegia. Unilateral cerebral lesions do not cause upper motor neuron lesions of most cranial nerves because of the compensation provided by bilateral cortical innervation.

    **E**  **True**  Cortical sensory loss involves two-point discrimination, joint position sense and stereognosis. Children with spastic hemiplegia may also have an homonymous hemianopia.

# PAPER N
## QUESTIONS

**N1** **Regarding syndromes associated with imprinting:**
- **A** imprinting is described as the phenomenon of a gene or region of a chromosome being more likely to be expressed when inherited from one parent than the other.
- **B** Prader–Willi syndrome is due to a paternal deletion of chromosome 15q11–13 in 70% of cases.
- **C** Angelman syndrome is due to a paternal deletion of chromosome 15q11–13 in 70% of cases.
- **D** Beckwith–Wiedemann syndrome (BWS) results from both copies of the gene on chromosome 11p being inactivated.
- **E** uniparental disomy occurs when an individual inherits both chromosomes from one parent.

**N2** **Chickenpox (varicella) is characterized by:**
- **A** increased clinical severity if the source of infection is a sibling.
- **B** sequential appearance of different crops of vesicles.
- **C** possible development of ataxia.
- **D** appearance of the rash on the third day of the illness.
- **E** causation of Kaposi's varicelliform eruption in children with eczema.

**N3** **Neuroblastoma:**
- **A** is the commonest extracranial solid tumour in children.
- **B** has a worse prognosis when it presents in infancy.
- **C** always leads to an increase in urine catecholamine excretion.
- **D** may be confused with orbital rhabdomyosarcoma.
- **E** may present with opsoclonus.

**N4** **The following are general features of primary immunodeficiencies (PID):**
- **A** the overall incidence is very similar to that of phenylketonuria.
- **B** failure to thrive is a commonly associated feature.
- **C** bone marrow transplantation is indicated in all T and B lymphocyte function deficiencies.
- **D** PID should be suspected in any child who has had two (or more) invasive bacterial infections.

**E** PID commonly presents with infections of increasing severity.

**N5**   In Henoch–Schönlein purpura (HSP):
- **A**   the platelet count is normal.
- **B**   renal involvement may lead to hypertension.
- **C**   abdominal pain is usually due to gastritis.
- **D**   the initial presenting symptom may be arthropathy.
- **E**   the rash is due to vasculitis.

**N6**   Maternal serum alpha fetoprotein (AFP) measured at 12 weeks' gestation:
- **A**   if normal then neural tube defects are excluded.
- **B**   is increased in twin pregnancies.
- **C**   is reduced in Turner syndrome.
- **D**   is increased in Down syndrome.
- **E**   AFP is the main blood protein fraction in the first trimester.

**N7**   The following statements regarding asthma in childhood are correct:
- **A**   in an acute exacerbation, a $P_{CO_2}$ of 5.8 kPa is more reassuring than one of 3.0 kPa.
- **B**   smooth muscle is not present in the bronchioles of a 3-month-old child.
- **C**   around 15–20% of children are affected at some time in their childhood.
- **D**   most childhood asthma deaths are preventable.
- **E**   sodium cromoglycate is normally given on a once-daily basis.

**N8**   The Mental Health Act (1983):
- **A**   is applicable to the 14–18-year age group.
- **B**   allows compulsory admission for assessment for 28 days.
- **C**   refers to the Children Act regarding the handling of children aged 10–14 years.
- **D**   a 72-hour detention order can only be obtained by a consultant psychiatrist or a 'nominated deputy'.
- **E**   requires the making of a treatment order for medication to be given against a patient's will.

**N9**   Secondary nocturnal enuresis may be associated with:
- **A**   sexual abuse.
- **B**   chronic renal failure.
- **C**   absence seizures ('petit mal').
- **D**   histiocytosis X.
- **E**   hypothyroidism.

**N10**   The following treatments can result in hypokalaemia:
- **A**   intravenous Darrow's solution.
- **B**   intravenous aminophylline.

C    intravenous insulin and dextrose.
D    cessation of long-term systemic steroid therapy.
E    laxative abuse.

**N11**   **A 2-year-old boy presents with three separate episodes of fever, coughing and patchy opacities on chest X-ray in the last 12 months. The following steps are indicated:**
A    X-ray of frontal sinuses.
B    prophylactic penicillin V for 12 months.
C    BCG vaccination.
D    sweat test.
E    serum immunoglobulin estimation.

**N12**   **Cystic fibrosis may present in the following ways:**
A    meconium ileus.
B    feeding problems in the first two years of life.
C    hyponatraemia during a heat wave.
D    'asthma' combined with 'toddler diarrhoea'.
E    erythema nodosum.

**N13**   **Referral to child psychiatry should be seriously considered in:**
A    an 8-year-old boy who is a persistent bully.
B    a 14-year-old girl who has taken an overdose of contraceptive pills after a row with her best friend at school.
C    a 12-year-old girl who has missed 2 months of school with abdominal pain.
D    an 8-year-old girl who teachers say always looks sad.
E    a 10-year-old boy who is markedly reluctant to return home after a short hospital admission.

**N14**   **Ataxia telangiectasia has the following features:**
A    raised serum alpha fetoprotein.
B    defective IgA mediated immunity.
C    X-linked recessive inheritance.
D    telangiectasia of the conjunctivae in the first year of life.
E    increased risk of acute lymphoblastic leukaemia.

**N15**   **Hereditary spherocytosis:**
A    is usually inherited in a sex-linked recessive fashion.
B    may necessitate exchange transfusion in the neonatal period.
C    should routinely be treated by splenectomy in infancy.
D    cannot be diagnosed in asymptomatic patients.
E    may be complicated by gall stones.

**N16**   **Regarding malaria:**
A    it is transmitted by sporozoites carried by mosquitoes.
B    red blood cells infected with *P. falciparum* adhere to vascular endothelium.

    **C** chloroquine is the drug of choice in a Caucasian child with falciparum malaria recently returned from a holiday in East Africa.
    **D** children with sickle cell anaemia are relatively resistant to malaria.
    **E** exchange transfusion should be considered for cases of severe falciparum malaria with parasite counts exceeding 10%.

**N17** **Nitric oxide (NO):**
    **A** stimulates production of cyclic AMP.
    **B** if used by the inhaled route produces a fall in systemic vascular resistance.
    **C** is produced by the body.
    **D** can be useful in the management of persistent fetal circulation.
    **E** increases the production of surfactant.

**N18** **Recognized neonatal complications of maternal systemic lupus erythematosus include:**
    **A** erythematous rash.
    **B** polycythaemia.
    **C** congenital heart block.
    **D** atrial fibrillation.
    **E** neutropenia.

**N19** **In a 5-year-old boy without haematuria, hypertension or renal failure who presents with nephrotic syndrome:**
    **A** a trial of up to one month of prednisolone 60 mg/m² is justified without performing a renal biopsy.
    **B** penicillin V is indicated if a child has an upper respiratory tract infection.
    **C** a low C3 is suggestive of steroid sensitive nephrotic syndrome.
    **D** after successful treatment with prednisolone relapses are unlikely.
    **E** the final outcome for renal function is likely to be normal.

**N20** **The following statements regarding the anatomy of the respiratory tract are true:**
    **A** the blood supply to the bronchi is derived from the systemic circulation.
    **B** lymphatic drainage of the parietal pleura is to the mediastinal lymph nodes.
    **C** the number of alveoli increases 10-fold from birth to adult life.
    **D** the diaphragm is innervated from the 3rd, 4th and 5th cervical segments.
    **E** the right main bronchus is longer than the left.

# PAPER N
## ANSWERS

**N1**  **A**  **True**

    **B**  **True**    This includes cytogenetically visible and submicroscopic deletions.

    **C**  **False**    Angelman syndrome is due to a *maternal* deletion of chromosome 15q11–13 in 70% of cases.

    **D**  **False**    BWS is due to activation of both copies of the gene, the maternal copy normally being silent. Activation of the maternal copy or alternatively duplication of the paternal copy can both result in BWS.

    **E**  **True**

**N2**  **A**  **True**    This is thought to be due to an increased load of virus at the onset of the infection. In addition, the incubation period may be shortened (from c. 15 days to c. 10 days).

    **B**  **True**    This 'cropping' of vesicles is pathognomonic of chickenpox and used to be used to differentiate it from the now obsolete smallpox.

    **C**  **True**    Encephalitis may occur within the first week of the illness and this has an especial predilection for the cerebellum.

    **D**  **False**    The rash appears on the first day of the illness.

    **E**  **False**    Kaposi's varicelliform eruption is caused by herpes simplex virus. This is a troublesome and occasionally fatal condition.

**N3**  **A**  **True**

    **B**  **False**    The prognosis is better in infants, worse in children over 2 years of age.

    **C**  **False**    Urine catecholamines are raised in most but not all cases.

    **D**  **True**    Neuroblastoma commonly presents with apparent orbital bruising and proptosis, and the differential diagnosis includes an orbital rhabdomyosarcoma and non-accidental injury.

**E   True**   Opsoclonus (rapid random eye movements) and ataxia are recognized symptoms of neuroblastoma ('dancing eyes, dancing feet').

**N4   A   True**   The figure is around 1:14 000 live births.

**B   True**

**C   False**   For instance, X-linked agammaglobulinaemia is well treated with immunoglobulin replacement and the risks of bone marrow transplantation would therefore be too great.

**D   True**   For example, an episode of bacterial meningitis followed by a bacterial pneumonia.

**E   True**

**N5   A   True**   The purpuric rash in HSP is due to vasculitis of small blood vessels, not thrombocytopenia.

**B   True**   HSP can cause an acute nephritic illness which may lead to hypertension. It can also cause nephrotic syndrome.

**C   False**   The abdominal pain (which with the arthropathy and purpura comprises the classical triad of HSP) is due to bleeding into the gastrointestinal mucosa. This may even lead to intussusception. Steroids appear to suppress the alimentary pathology while having no effect on the purpura or renal pathology.

**D   True**
**E   True**

**N6   A   False**   AFP *may* be raised in neural tube defects but a normal level does not exclude this group of conditions. *Closed* neural tube defects do not raise maternal AFP.

**B   True**

**C   False**   AFP can be *increased* in Turner syndrome.

**D   False**   AFP is characteristically *reduced* in Down syndrome.

**E   True**

**N7   A   False**   In the evolution of an increasingly severe attack, the $Pco_2$ initially drops to low levels due to compensatory hyperventilation. As the attack worsens, the $Pco_2$ rises, passing through normal levels to raised levels, which reflect generalized alveolar hypoventilation. Thus, normal levels are more worrying than low levels in the context of an acute attack.

**B** **False**

**C** **True** The prevalence of childhood asthma appears to be rising steadily, and 15–20% is a best guess for clinical asthma at present.

**D** **True** In common with studies in adult medicine, it is thought that around 80% of childhood asthma deaths could be prevented (mainly by giving parents crisis packs which include crash courses of steroids and instructions on when to use them).

**E** **False** One of the disadvantages of this prophylactic drug is the need to give it four times a day.

**N8** **A** **True** The Act is applicable to children and adolescents as no lower age limit is stipulated. It could be invoked more often than it is with teenagers who are serious suicide risks.

**B** **True**

**C** **False** The Children Act was drafted in 1989!

**D** **True**

**E** **False** Treatment can be given under common law where behaviour represents an immediate risk to self or others as a result of mental disorder.

**N9** **A** **True** Secondary nocturnal enuresis (a relapse in bedwetting in a child who has been dry for some time) can be due to emotional disturbance, and sexual abuse is naturally a potent cause of this.

**B** **True** Chronic renal failure will cause an osmotic polyuria which will increase the chance of bedwetting.

**C** **False** Generalized major seizures may present as secondary bedwetting, but one would not expect this in simple absence seizures.

**D** **True** As a result of polyuria secondary to diabetes insipidus.

**E** **False**

**N10** **A** **False** Darrow's solution was designed to *replace* potassium in the treatment of gastro-enteritis. It contains 30–35 mmol of potassium per litre. This is too much for rapid treatment of dehydration, and in developing countries it is usually used at half-strength diluted with 5% dextrose.

**B  True**  The three main types of drugs for the treatment of acute asthma (aminophylline, $B_2$ agonists and steroids) all cause hypokalaemia. This can be a practical problem especially if the attack is preceded by long-term oral theophyllines, and if hydrocortisone is used instead of prednisolone (as it loses more potassium for the same anti-inflammatory effect).

**C  True**  Intravenous insulin and dextrose are recognized as one of the emergency treatments for hyperkalaemia (together with calcium gluconate, resonium and dialysis). In the management of diabetic ketoacidosis, hypokalaemia is almost universally found after the first few hours unless potassium replacement is started early.

**D  False**  Cessation of long-term steroid therapy will cause an Addisonian crisis with hyponatraemia and *hyperkalaemia*.

**E  True**  Chronic laxative abuse (e.g. in teenage girls with eating disorders) can cause hypokalaemia through loss of potassium through the diarrhoeal fluid.

**N11  A  False**  While there is an association between sinusitis and bronchiectasis (due to ciliary dyskinesia), the sinuses are so poorly developed at this age that X-ray is of little value.

**B  False**  While there may be an underlying immunodeficiency in this case, further evaluation is necessary before decisions on therapy. In any case, it is unlikely that penicillin V would be the antibiotic of choice in view of its narrow spectrum.

**C  False**  Mantoux testing might be a useful investigation at this stage as the child might be suffering from primary TB. However, BCG vaccination would be irrational, and might turn out to be positively contraindicated if the child turns out to have an immunodeficiency.

**D  True**

**E  True**

**N12  A  True**  All cases of meconium ileus should be followed up and have repeated sweat tests.

**B  False**  Children with cystic fibrosis may present with failure to thrive but this is due to malabsorption not poor intake. Typically, children with cystic fibrosis have good appetites.

**C   True**   Full-blown 'heat exhaustion' with circulatory collapse may occur in tropical heat, due to increased loss of salt in sweat. Salt supplements should be considered as a preventive measure.

**D   True**   Both asthma and toddler diarrhoea are very common in the childhood population, and not all children with cystic fibrosis fail to thrive.

**E   False**

**N13   A   True**   Persistent bullying is pathological and can be regarded as a form of conduct disorder. It carries a poor prognosis, being strongly associated with later delinquency and criminal behaviour.

**B   True**   While this episode sounds trivial both in terms of the trigger and the degree of danger, all episodes of teenage self-harm deserve proper assessment, as often deeper problems are revealed.

**C   False**   Neither the length of school loss nor the fact that the pain is abdominal is an indication per se for psychiatric referral. The old idea that 90% of recurrent abdominal pain is non-organic, therefore functional, therefore psychosomatic, is best regarded as a myth, especially since the recognition that most of these cases are probably abdominal migraine which is easy to treat medically.

**D   True**   Persistent sadness at any age but especially in a latency age child should always be taken seriously. Latency age children are very resilient and it takes a lot to make them sad.

**E   True**   This should be taken extremely seriously as it is most unnatural and is suggestive of a significant degree of emotional abuse and deprivation at home.

**N14   A   True**

**B   True**

**C   False**   Inheritance is autosomal recessive.

**D   False**   Telangiectases do not appear till the age of 4–5 years. They also occur on the neck and shoulders.

**E   True**   The risk is about 10%. The ataxia associated with the condition becomes increasingly severe throughout childhood.

**N15   A   False**   Most cases are inherited in an autosomal dominant fashion.

**B**    **True**    It may present in the neonatal period with severe unconjugated hyperbilirubinaemia (due to haemolysis) necessitating exchange transfusion. It is difficult to establish the diagnosis in the first few weeks of life. Most cases are diagnosed as a result of the positive family history.

**C**    **False**    Splenectomy is very rarely required in infancy. Not every case requires splenectomy and it should not be resorted to unless absolutely essential because of the degree of immunodeficiency that results from splenectomy.

**D**    **False**    Most cases will have splenomegaly, but otherwise they may not be clinically jaundiced or anaemic. Such cases can still be diagnosed definitely by an abnormal osmotic fragility test.

**E**    **True**    These are due to excess production of bile pigments as a result of haemolysis.

**N16**    **A**    **True**

**B**    **True**    In addition to mechanical obstruction of capillaries by schizont-infected cells, the latter have been shown to actively adhere to vascular endothelium.

**C**    **False**    There is a high incidence of chloroquine resistance in East Africa, and therefore the first choice in this potentially life-threatening condition should be either a sulphonamide–pyrimethamine combination (e.g. Fansidar) or quinine.

**D**    **False**    Children with sickle cell *trait* (HbAS) are relatively resistant to malaria, but children with full sickle cell anaemia (HbSS) are at *increased* risk of malaria compared with normal children.

**E**    **True**

**N17**    **A**    **False**    Nitric oxide activates guanidyl cyclase and thereby stimulates cyclic guanidyl monophosphate (GMP) production, not cAMP.

**B**    **False**    Inhaled nitric oxide is increasingly being used because of its ability to act as a potent pulmonary vasodilator, without producing a fall in systemic vascular resistance. This is because it is inactivated in the lung.

**C**    **True**    Interestingly, the ability to produce nitric oxide is distributed widely in the animal kingdom and clearly goes back a long way in evolutionary terms.

**D**    **True**    See (B).

**E**    **False**

**N18**  **A**  **True**

    **B**  **False**

    **C**  **True**    Mechanism unknown.

    **D**  **False**

    **E**  **True**

**N19**  **A**  **True**    The most likely diagnosis in this situation is steroid sensitive nephrotic syndrome and a renal biopsy is not justified unless a month of high-dose steroids fails to induce a remission. More than 97% of children with steroid sensitive nephrotic syndrome will respond within a month.

    **B**  **False**    Because children with nephrotic syndrome lose antibodies as well as albumin they are susceptible to pneumococcal infection. Twice-daily penicillin V prophylaxis should therefore be given to protect against this. URTIs commonly provoke relapses in children with steroid sensitive nephrotic syndrome, but these are usually viral in origin.

    **C**  **False**    The C3 is normal in steroid sensitive nephrotic syndrome and a low value suggests another diagnosis such as mesangiocapillary glomerulonephritis or systemic lupus. In this situation a renal biopsy is indicated to establish the diagnosis.

    **D**  **False**    The majority of children with steroid sensitive nephrotic syndrome relapse, commonly in association with viral infections. They then need further steroid treatment.

    **E**  **True**    Though most children have a relapsing course, virtually all outgrow the tendency and are eventually left with completely normal kidney function.

**N20**  **A**  **True**    Via the aorta and intercostal arteries.

    **B**  **False**    The parietal pleura has a similar lymphatic drainage to the ribs and chest wall, i.e. to superficial glands in the neck.

    **C**  **True**

    **D**  **True**    The diaphragm arises from these segments embryologically; this is why pain from diaphragmatic irritation is referred to the shoulder tip, and why a stitch is often felt in the supraclavicular area on exertion.

    **E**  **False**

# PAPER O
## QUESTIONS

**O1** **Regarding childhood diabetes:**
A diabetic children should receive less carbohydrate than non-diabetic children.
B insulin dosage should be increased over the week of an activity holiday.
C when a newly diagnosed diabetic is first discharged from hospital, the dose of insulin should be reduced.
D if a child vomits continuously for 72 hours, insulin therapy should be withheld until oral intake recommences.
E a large carbohydrate binge can tip a child into ketoacidosis.

**O2** **The following statements concerning infection in children receiving cytotoxic treatment are correct:**
A measles may lead to fatal encephalitis.
B blood cultures reveal the causative agent in the majority of children with systemic fungal infection.
C fever in a neutropenic child should not be treated with antibiotics until a positive culture result has been obtained.
D *Pneumocystis carinii* pneumonia (PCP) should be treated with high-dose erythromycin.
E all routine childhood immunizations may be given safely.

**O3** **Regarding epilepsy in children:**
A as a group, children with epilepsy show a high prevalence of psychiatric disorders.
B seizures are characteristic of disease affecting cerebral white matter.
C the incidence of epilepsy is higher in the neonatal period than at any later age.
D half of all cases of epilepsy have presented by the age of 8.
E idiopathic neonatal seizures have a reasonably good prognosis.

**O4** **Untreated phenylketonuria causes:**
A eczema.
B salaam spasms.
C blue eyes.
D Tourette syndrome.
E heart defects.

O5    **The following conditions can cause the combination of abdominal pain and a bloody stool in childhood:**
A    Meckel's diverticulum.
B    abdominal migraine.
C    Henoch–Schönlein purpura (HSP).
D    pelviureteric junction (PUJ) obstruction.
E    intussusception.

O6    **The likelihood of a child with febrile convulsions developing later epilepsy is influenced by:**
A    the presence of a family history of febrile convulsions.
B    a history of partial febrile convulsions.
C    the onset of febrile convulsions before 12 months.
D    the number of seizures occurring within a single febrile illness.
E    the duration of the febrile seizures.

O7    **Antibiotic prophylaxis against bacterial endocarditis is required in the following types of heart disease in children:**
A    atrial septal defect (ostium secundum type).
B    bicuspid aortic valve.
C    dilated cardiomyopathy.
D    hypertrophic obstructive cardiomyopathy (HOCM).
E    coarctation of the aorta.

O8    **The following are features of Prader–Willi syndrome:**
A    obesity.
B    large hands and feet.
C    hypotonia in infancy.
D    normal fertility.
E    associated with a deletion of maternal chromosome.

O9    **The following kidney conditions are inherited in the manner described:**
A    cystinosis by dominant inheritance.
B    infantile polycystic kidney disease (PCKD) by recessive inheritance.
C    adult polycystic kidney disease by X-linked recessive inheritance.
D    Alport syndrome by dominant inheritance.
E    bloody diarrhoea plus haemolytic uraemic syndrome (D + HUS) by recessive inheritance.

O10    **Parvovirus B19 infection:**
A    is the cause of herpangina.
B    in pregnancy can lead to hydrops fetalis.
C    causes a rash within the first 2–3 days of the illness.
D    causes pleurodynia.
E    can cause aplastic crises.

**O11** **The following is true of Kawasaki disease:**
A   thrombocytopenia is a common feature.
B   early aspirin therapy reduces the risk of coronary aneurysms.
C   Nikolsky's sign is usually positive.
D   the characteristic peeling of the fingers usually occurs in the first week.
E   mortality is 1–2%

**O12** **The pupillary light reflex depends upon the integrity of:**
A   the optic nerve.
B   the lateral geniculate nuclei.
C   the occipital cortex.
D   the medial longitudinal fasciculus.
E   the IIIrd (oculomotor) cranial nerve.

**O13** **The following statements regarding paediatric respiratory infections are true:**
A   mycoplasma infections are an important cause of community acquired pneumonia.
B   the pneumococcus characteristically causes a patchy bilateral bronchopneumonia.
C   the treatment of choice for an aspergilloma is surgical.
D   vitamin A treatment should be considered in the management of a malnourished child with a giant-cell pneumonia.
E   penicillin remains the drug of choice in developing countries for the treatment of pneumonia.

**O14** **An 18-month-old child presents with fever, respiratory distress and clinical signs consistent with left lower lobe consolidation and a large effusion on the same side. The following statements are correct:**
A   the combination of penicillin and flucloxacillin would cover the pathogens most likely to give this picture.
B   if a tuberculous origin was suspected, a Heaf test would be the investigation of choice.
C   after 5 days of intravenous antibiotics, a diagnostic tap of the effusion is unlikely to give useful information.
D   in the presence of an unremitting fever after 1 week of broad spectrum antibiotics, a malignant cause is the most likely aetiology.
E   the presence of a phlyctenular conjunctivitis would considerably influence the management.

**O15** **The following are true concerning growth:**
A   any child whose height falls from the 75th centile at birth to the 10th centile at 2 years of age should be fully investigated.
B   the height velocity around the time of puberty is greater than at any other time.

C   the spleen is larger at the age of 12 years than in
adulthood.
D   the earliest sign of puberty in males is enlargement of the
penis.
E   at the age of 5 years, the brain is about 50% of its adult
weight.

**O16   The following may be of diagnostic significance in the
assessment of a hypotonic neonate:**
A   serum creatine kinase.
B   teenage parents with a strong aura of 'social problems'
around them.
C   relative sparing of muscles of facial expression.
D   karyotype analysis.
E   poor feeding.

**O17   The following may be associated with sudden bilateral visual
deterioration:**
A   growth failure.
B   uncomplicated papilloedema.
C   migraine.
D   painful eye movements.
E   loss of smell.

**O18   The facial nerve:**
A   subserves no cutaneous sensory function.
B   gives a motor supply to the inner ear.
C   controls movement of the anterior two thirds of the
tongue.
D   carries parasympathetic fibres to the salivary glands.
E   innervates platysma.

**O19   Cornelia de Lange syndrome is characterized by:**
A   gastro-oesophageal reflux.
B   moderate to severe learning difficulties.
C   low hairline.
D   beaked nose.
E   an increased incidence of congenital heart disease.

**O20   In a 5-year-old with hypertension:**
A   systolic blood pressure is a more useful measure than
diastolic.
B   blood pressure measurements should be made with a cuff
no more than two thirds of the length of the upper arm.
C   a family history of 'essential' hypertension is likely to be
important.
D   the initial imaging investigations would include an IVU.
E   there is greater than a 90% chance of it having a renal
cause.

# PAPER O
## ANSWERS

**O1 A False**   Diabetic children have exactly the same nutritional requirements as non-diabetic children, and they should both be given similar advice on 'healthy eating'. However, it is especially desirable for diabetic children to take most of their carbohydrate in complex rather than refined form.

**B False**   The child will be at increased risk of hypoglycaemic attacks with the increased activity. Carbohydrate intake should be increased and insulin dosage either kept constant or slightly reduced.

**C True**   The child is at risk of 'hypos' for two reasons: (i) he/she will be more active on return home; (ii) there is a tendency for dosage requirements to fall after initial stabilization.

**D False**   A recipe for death. All diabetic children need insulin every day for the rest of their lives. Any infection increases the need for insulin. Naturally, the child should be given calories in the form of IV dextrose over this period.

**E False**   A common myth. If the child is well and taking his/her regular insulin, an extra carbohydrate load will simply cause hyperglycaemia and glycosuria without ketosis.

**O2 A True**   Measles encephalitis is rare in immunocompetent children, but much commoner and frequently fatal in immunocompromised subjects.

**B False**   It is relatively rare to make a positive microbiological diagnosis of fungal infection from blood cultures — the diagnosis and decision to treat is therefore best made on a high index of clinical suspicion.

**C False**   Failure to treat empirically a febrile neutropenic child with broad spectrum antibiotics runs a high risk of a fatal outcome from rapidly progressive overwhelming sepsis.

|   | **D** | **False** | PCP should be treated with high-dose cotrimoxazole. |
|---|---|---|---|
|   | **E** | **False** | All live attenuated vaccines (e.g. oral polio, MMR) must be totally avoided until at least six months after the end of all chemotherapy (longer for children who have received a bone marrow transplant). |
| **O3** | **A** | **True** | Rutter's Isle of Wight study showed that children with 'uncomplicated' epilepsy had a 4-fold higher risk of psychiatric disorder, rising to 10-fold if there was an associated neurological disorder. |
|   | **B** | **False** | Seizures are a result of cortical (grey matter) disease. In general, white matter disease tends to present with motor (pyramidal or cerebellar) signs. |
|   | **C** | **True** | Convulsions in the neonatal period affect 125 cases per 100 000 and this is higher than at any other age. The age-related incidence remains high until 4 or 5, then falls through later childhood. |
|   | **D** | **False** | Only 50% of cases of epilepsy have presented by the age of 15–16. |
|   | **E** | **True** | While 'idiopathic' is often a diagnosis made by exclusion and in retrospect, the prognosis in such cases is often excellent. Naturally neonatal seizures due to hypoxic–ischaemic encephalopathy, neonatal infection or congenital CNS anomalies have a far worse prognosis. |
| **O4** | **A** | **True** | Phenylketonuria is very rare and occurs in 1 in 10–20 000 births. It should be picked up by the Guthrie screening test so it should be exceedingly rare to see an untreated case. Eczema is more common in affected children, who are also likely to have blue eyes and fair hair. |
|   | **B** | **True** | Affected children usually present with infantile spasms and/or developmental delay in the first 6–12 months of age. |
|   | **C** | **True** | See (A) |
|   | **D** | **False** | |
|   | **E** | **False** | |
| **O5** | **A** | **True** | Peptic ulceration of a Meckel's diverticulum can cause both abdominal pain and lower gastrointestinal bleeding. |
|   | **B** | **False** | |

C **True** Abdominal pain is one of the cardinal three features of HSP (the others being a purpuric rash and joint pains). Bleeding per rectum can result from either simple bleeding into the wall of the bowel or else an actual intussusception.

D **False**

E **True** Ideally, intussusception should be suspected and diagnosed clinically *before* the passage of a bloody stool. The suggestive feature on the history is episodic screaming over a period of hours.

O6 A **False** A family history of febrile convulsions predisposes only to febrile convulsions, not epilepsy.

B **True** A partial (or focal) febrile convulsion is by definition a 'complicated' as opposed to a 'simple' febrile convulsion, and as such carries a 10% risk of subsequent epilepsy.

C **False** Onset before the age of 6 months would carry the 10% risk mentioned above, but before 12 months is unremarkable.

D **True** Occurrence of more than one seizure in a single febrile illness increases the risk.

E **True** Duration of over 15 minutes is defined as a 'complicated' seizure (see above).

O7 A **False** This is virtually the only significant structural heart lesion that has been shown not to be at increased risk of endocarditis. The negligible risk is presumably due to the low degree of turbulence involved.

B **True** Current orthodoxy advises prophylaxis in known cases of this condition. However, the risk must be fairly low as most of the 1% of the population with bicuspid aortic valves remain undiagnosed and do not receive prophylaxis.

C **False**

D **True**

E **True**

O8 A **True** After initial failure to thrive, children with this condition become grossly obese, especially during adolescence. There is an increased risk of diabetes mellitus as a result.

| | | |
|---|---|---|
| **B** | **False** | The hands and feet are relatively small. Large hands and feet (and macrocephaly) are a feature of Soto syndrome (cerebral gigantism). |
| **C** | **True** | |
| **D** | **False** | Hypogonadism is a cardinal feature of this condition. |
| **E** | **False** | Prader–Willi syndrome is caused by a deletion of *paternal* chromosome 15q11–13. A very similar deletion of a *maternal* chromosome 15 gives rise to Angelman syndrome. This is known by geneticists by the term 'imprinting'. |

**O9**

| | | |
|---|---|---|
| **A** | **False** | Cystinosis is recessively inherited. Without transplantation few patients survive into their second decade so dominant inheritance is not possible. |
| **B** | **True** | Most children with infantile PCKD develop end-stage renal failure in infancy or early childhood, so dominant inheritance is not possible. |
| **C** | **False** | Adult PCKD is *dominantly* inherited through a gene on chromosome 16. Up to 10% of cases are new mutations. Most children inheriting the gene have normal kidney ultrasound appearances at birth but develop cysts with time. Renal failure is very rare before the third or fourth decade. |
| **D** | **False** | Alport syndrome is inherited by an X-linked recessive pattern. Thus, most women with Alport syndrome merely have microscopic haematuria and a small amount of proteinuria, but because of Lyonization of the X chromosome approximately 5% behave like males with Alport syndrome. Boys with Alport syndrome usually develop proteinuria and macroscopic haematuria before the age of 5 and reach end-stage renal failure at a median age of 18 years. Deafness is almost universal and parallels the deterioration of renal function. The link between the ear and kidney is that Alport patients fail to produce normal Type IV collagen which is present in the basement membrane of the glomerulus and the cochlea. |
| **E** | **False** | D + HUS is an infectious illness caused by a verotoxin-producing organism. There are however some inherited forms of HUS *without* diarrhoea (D – HUS). |

**O10**

| | | |
|---|---|---|
| **A** | **False** | Herpangina is caused by Coxsackie A infection. |
| **B** | **True** | |

| | C | **False** | The most common effect of parvovirus B19 infection is erythema infectiosum, which causes a febrile illness for one week before the characteristic rash appears (slapped cheek syndrome). |
|---|---|---|---|

    **D**  **False**  Pleurodynia (Bornholm disease) is caused by Coxsackie B infection.

    **E**  **True**  This is especially likely in children with chronic haemolytic anaemia (e.g. spherocytosis, haemoglobinopathies).

**O11**  **A**  **False**  Kawasaki disease is an important and probably underdiagnosed condition in which 30% of children develop aneurysms of their coronary arteries with a subsequent risk of myocardial infarction. Ideally the diagnosis should be made clinically in the first 10 days as IV immunoglobulin at this stage has been shown to reduce the incidence of coronary aneurysms. Unfortunately, the classical peeling of the fingertips does not occur till the third week. An *increased* platelet count in the second week is usual and can be a vital clue in considering the diagnosis.

    **B**  **False**  Aspirin is given for its antiplatelet effects to reduce the risk of coronary thrombosis in those with aneurysms. It is not thought to reduce the actual incidence of aneurysms.

    **C**  **False**  This sign only occurs in conditions like staphylococcal scalded skin syndrome or epidermolysis bullosa, and consists of showing that the epidermis can be detached from the dermis by pressure.

    **D**  **False**  See (A).

    **E**  **True**

**O12**  **A**  **True**  The sensory component of the pupillary light reflex is conveyed from the retina via the optic nerve to the chiasm. Here the nerve decussates and conveys impulses to both optic tracts and both lateral geniculate nuclei. Here some fibres are relayed to both Edinger–Westphal nuclei (the IIIrd nerve nucleus), and complete the motor component of the light reflex. This bilaterality is responsible for the consensuality of the normal pupillary reflex.

    **B**  **True**  See above.

C  **False**  A patient can be cortically blind due to occipital cortex destruction but will still have intact pupillary reflexes.

D  **False**  The medial longitudinal fasciculus is involved in controlling conjugate eye movements.

E  **True**  See above.

O13  A  **True**  This statement is true for both children and adults. Mycoplasma causes a primary atypical pneumonia with a troublesome cough, basal crepitations and patchy interstitial shadowing on chest X-ray. It can occur in mini-epidemics in communities and within families. Erythromycin is the treatment of choice.

B  **False**  The pneumococcus most often causes a classic lobar pneumonia.

C  **True**

D  **True**  In developing countries giant-cell pneumonia due to measles has been shown to have an improved prognosis if vitamin A supplements are added to the other treatments.

E  **False**  The WHO has recommended cotrimoxazole as the drug of choice for pneumonia in developing countries on the grounds of good oral absorption, broadness of spectrum and relative cheapness.

O14  A  **False**  This combination would not cover *Haemophilus influenzae* or *Klebsiella pneumoniae*.

B  **False**  The Heaf test is a screening test for use in the community. The Mantoux test (starting at 1:10 000 → 1:1000) gives more helpful information in the individual case.

C  **False**  Antibiotics penetrate poorly into pleural effusions and empyemas. A positive culture may be obtained if (a) the empyema is encysted or (b) the wrong antibiotics are being used.

D  **False**  An encysted empyema would be a far commoner explanation.

E  **True**  This would suggest primary pulmonary tuberculosis.

O15  A  **False**  If the midparental height is around the 10th centile this finding is probably entirely benign. Growth in the first 2 years of life is more a reflection of intrauterine and infant nutrition, and it is only after this that the child reveals his/her true growth potential.

**B  False**  Reference to a standard height velocity chart reveals a height velocity in the first 2 years of life that is 2–3 times that achieved at puberty.

**C  True**  In common with all lymphoid tissue, the spleen regresses significantly in size as adulthood is approached.

**D  False**  The earliest sign is enlargement of the testes which occurs in response to pituitary gonadotrophins.

**E  False**  By the age of 5 the brain has already attained 90% of its adult weight.

**O16  A  True**  A high serum CK suggests muscular dystrophy, which at this age may be congenital (autosomal recessive) muscular dystrophy rather than Duchenne dystrophy.

**B  True**  Maternal use in the last trimester of either narcotic drugs or benzodiazepines could be responsible for the infant being floppy.

**C  True**  Relative sparing of the muscles of facial expression is characteristic of Werdnig–Hoffmann disease (severe neonatal onset form of spinal muscular dystrophy).

**D  True**  Prader–Willi syndrome is an important condition presenting with neonatal hypotonia. The feeding is characteristically disproportionately affected. The diagnosis can be confirmed by demonstrating the 15q deletion syndrome.

**E  True**  See (D).

**O17  A  True**  The gradual onset of a bitemporal hemianopia (due to craniopharyngioma) may go relatively unnoticed until eventually the macula is involved when it will suddenly be apparent.

**B  False**  Mild tunnel vision is seldom noticed by the patient, and only complications (such as haemorrhage) will present with sudden visual deterioration.

**C  True**  Migraine can present with a wide range of visual phenomena including transient blindness.

**D  True**  Painful eye movements are suggestive of optic neuritis which can present with bilateral central scotomata.

**E  False**  In adults, slow growing olfactory meningiomas can cause visual disturbance, but the deterioration is gradual and unilateral.

**O18**  **A**  **False**  Although predominantly motor, the VIIth cranial nerve has a clinically important cutaneous sensory supply to the skin of the external auditory canal (from the vagus). Vesicles in this area combined with a facial palsy are diagnostic of the Ramsay Hunt syndrome (geniculate herpes zoster).

  **B**  **False**  *Middle* ear, nerve to the stapedius.

  **C**  **False**  The VIIth nerve conveys *sensory* fibres (taste) (via the chorda tympani) from the anterior two thirds of the tongue. (The motor supply to the whole of the tongue is via the XIIth cranial nerve.)

  **D**  **True**

  **E**  **True**  The platysma is best thought of as a muscle of facial expression, even though it extends over the anterior surface of the neck to the upper chest.

**O19**  **A**  **True**  Cornelia de Lange syndrome (Amsterdam dwarfism) is a rare (1:40 000) condition characterized by short stature, distinctive facial features (thin 'pencilled' eyebrows, smooth philtrum, thin lips and low hairline) and mental retardation. In the classical form of the condition the latter is severe, in the milder form of the condition the retardation is mild to moderate. Gastro-oesophageal reflux occurs in 15–75% of cases and is frequently severe, often severe enough to require surgery.

  **B**  **True**  See (A).

  **C**  **True**  See (A).

  **D**  **False**

  **E**  **True**  In the severe form of the condition the incidence of congenital heart disease is around 20%, usually septal defects or Fallot's tetralogy.

**O20**  **A**  **True**  Systolic blood pressure can be measured with greater accuracy than diastolic whichever method is used, and can be measured by a wider range of methods than diastolic, including palpation of the radial artery and Doppler 'auscultation' over the radial artery. In young people with compliant arteries, systolic, mean and diastolic blood pressures all change in parallel to each other so the choice of best technique depends on ease and accuracy of measurement.

**B** **False** The largest cuff that can be fitted onto the upper arm and still allow blood pressure to be recorded will produce the most accurate value. Cuffs that are too small will produce an artificially high blood pressure reading. Sometimes two thirds of the length of the upper arm is too small and produces a false value.

**C** **False** Though 'tracking' of children's blood pressure does occur, such that children who will become adults with essential hypertension tend to drift upwards across the centiles, this correlation is very weak and is unlikely to be relevant in a 5-year-old.

**D** **False** Hypertension due to focal reflux nephropathy scarring is seen much earlier and more reliably using DMSA than intravenous urography. The persistent and intense nephrogram phase seen in an adult kidney with renal artery stenosis is virtually not seen in children.

**E** **True** The percentage of cases due to an identifiable renal cause is much higher in children than adults.

# SECTION 2

# A TACTICAL GUIDE
## HOW TO APPROACH CLINICAL EXAMINATIONS

### Introduction

Medical students are first taught how to *take* a clinical history and perform a clinical examination, and how to *record* their findings in the medical records. In the early stages of their undergraduate careers they are usually made to *present* their histories and examinations in full, presumably to encourage thoroughness. They then enter a period of clinical apprenticeship when they clerk more patients and increase their experience. Clinical teaching may continue to involve their presentation of cases, but if this is in the context of a business round, their presentation may often be cut short because it is too long-winded. By contrast, if a case is presented on a teaching round, this is usually quite a leisurely exercise in which the teacher frequently interrupts to ask questions of the group and to impart theoretical knowledge. Indeed, so much interruption may take place that the student is frequently spared the necessity of reaching the 'end' to which all else is but a 'means', namely the composition of a diagnostic summary which does justice to all the positive findings in the history and examination and which leads to a discussion of differential diagnosis. The net result of these tendencies is that students frequently find themselves somewhat unprepared for the rigours of the final clinical examinations. In these, time is severely limited, both for *taking* the history and performing the examination, for *thinking* about the case constructively and for subsequently *presenting* the case to the examiners. The long-winded 'medical student' approach is ill-fitted to this situation and many students find the abrupt transition traumatic.

The long and short case clinical examinations and vivas are well-designed instruments to test vital aspects of clinical skill and knowledge, and they have been preserved in these days of MCQs because they test qualities that cannot be tested in other ways. The qualities include the ability:

- to relate to patients
- to elicit a history that is diagnostically useful and not just a passive 'tape-recording' of the patient's words
- to use time intelligently and to concentrate on major rather than minor problems
- to elicit physical signs and to draw appropriate conclusions
- to present one's findings concisely and clearly, and to reach a reasoned differential diagnosis

- to discuss a topic intelligently and with balance
- to keep calm under pressure.

These are, of course, some of the ideal qualities we look for in our junior staff.

It is my belief that students are seldom told clearly enough of the need to progress from the 'medical student' approach to the 'practising doctor' approach. Examiners automatically judge final examination candidates by the latter standard, but no-one ever tells the students that the rules have changed! The effect is blurred by the fact that the vast majority of students pass their final examinations, and once qualified rapidly learn the facts of life doing busy clinical jobs. However, the time comes when postgraduate examinations have to be taken, and these usually carry a high failure rate. Frequently English graduates who 'have never failed an exam in their lives' come a cropper, and are chastened to find that the clinical method that sufficed for finals is now inadequate, and a more critical, thorough and polished approach is needed. Foreign graduates, often working in District General Hospitals with little teaching, similarly fail frequently. Despite all the knowledge that books can provide, they may fail in the clinicals simply because of faulty technique.

These guidelines are offered in the hope that they can help candidates to make the most of what knowledge they possess.

### Long case technique

*How to spend your time*

Some cases will have complex histories and few or no physical signs; others the reverse. Try to decide early on which type of case it is, and to spend the appropriate amount of time on each stage.

Make sure you are certain just how long you are allowed. Leave time to ascertain the *height* and *weight* of the child, find and use a centile chart, and test the urine when a sample is provided.

Most importantly, always leave 5–10 minutes free at the end to *think* about the case, to *structure* your presentation, and to *check or amplify important points in the history and examination*. When you've done all that, start trying to think what sort of questions the examiner might be likely to ask you concerning the case!

*Approaching the patient and parent*

The golden rule is **establish rapport first**, with both mother and child. **Don't** rush straight in with a stream of questions. Introduce yourself to the mother and *shake hands* with her (and the child when old enough). Allow yourself a minute or two to chat to the mother and child in a friendly sort of way — it is time well spent; e.g. 'I'm awfully sorry to bother you, you must find this all a bit boring. How many doctors have you seen already? I hope they've been nice to him. Do they pay you for coming? Gosh how awful, etc., etc. Well, my problem is I have to find out all about Jimmy here in a hurry, so forgive me if I rush through a lot of questions or cut you short at any time. Now could you tell me all about his illness?' Leave the last question open-ended so that the mother can tell you as much as possible spontaneously. Many will be practised historians and if you have approached them in a nice way they will be only too keen to help you as much as possible.

Naturally if you upset a mother or her child at any stage the mother may give you a grudging history with important gaps, and the child may be difficult to examine.

In the case of a chronic illness it is best to both *take* and *present* the history from the onset of the illness, rather than concentrating on a recent acute exacerbation and working backwards, thus relegating a lot of interesting material to the past medical history.

In an acute recent illness make sure you take the history *right up to the present day*, including the progress of all the symptoms in hospital, the details of and response to any treatments given, and an account of the investigations performed. The same would apply to a previous admission to hospital.

*Examination*

Try to stick to your usual routine and examine all systems in the usual order, but make sure you really *concentrate* on the affected system. Spend more time on it and cover every detail.

When you've finished the examination, and before your final 5–10 minute 'think', try asking the following questions (Pappworth):

1. *What have the doctors told you about this illness?*

   This is not cheating, but a perfectly fair question in any medical situation. In addition to confirming your diagnosis, the answers will often help to remind you of such areas as general management, genetic counselling, amniocentesis in future pregnancies, etc.

2. *What tests have they done on Jimmy?*

   Well doctor, they've stuck a needle in his back, and done a kidney X-ray, and sent him to an eye doctor and done a skin test on his arm, oh yes, and they've X-rayed his wrist because they think he's a bit small.

3. *What kind of treatment has he had?*

   Well doctor, they gave him some antibiotics in a drip but then they stopped them because they said it was a virus. Then they changed their minds and now he's on daily injections and some capsules that make his water red — I think they're against TB.

4. *What questions do the doctors keep asking?*

   Well they keep asking if he's ever been abroad, or drunk unpasteurized milk, or if anyone in the family has had TB, and they keep looking in his eyes and arguing about whether or not they can feel his spleen.

You can see how helpful these questions can be!

*Presenting the long case*

You are in charge! You can control the course of the whole presentation. Try to talk fluently and continuously for as long as possible, giving the examiner no chance to interrupt. Don't keep looking for encouragement to the examiner — he may remain in stony silence throughout.

Don't read from your notes — this puts the examiner straight to sleep. If you use notes at all, keep them brief and try to refer to them as little as possible. Try to establish and *maintain eye contact* with the examiner throughout. Try to inject some expression into your voice, and make your presentation as interesting as possible. Try to convey the impression that you are more than an automaton passively spewing out the history without any emotion. Thus, if the case is a tragic one (e.g. with four out of five children in the family suffering from cystic fibrosis) say so at the beginning. Similarly, if the previous medical management leaves something to be desired, allow your eyebrows to rise gently at the appropriate stage!

Ideally you want to cover all the following headings systematically and succinctly, ending up with time for discussion.

1. *A comprehensive introduction*

   This is most important. Briefly sketch the *essential details of the patient's life situation*, including age, position in family, father's occupation, where the family come from, racial origin where appropriate, etc. *Speak in sentences* and do not give unnecessary detail, e.g. the actual date of birth, address, etc. In addition, *paint the essential outline* of the patient's medical problems, thus letting the examiner know at an early stage that you have a good grasp of the case, and that all the rest of the presentation will be merely filling in the details. If the diagnosis is incontrovertible — e.g. diabetes mellitus, cystic fibrosis, asthma, etc. — mention it here. Otherwise, if the diagnosis is more open to debate, limit yourself to a more non-committal phraseology, e.g. 'a long-standing renal problem with a more recent acute respiratory problem'. Mention the reason why the patient is actually in hospital at the moment, e.g. recent acute exacerbation of chronic problem, or just brought in for the exam.

   (Evidence that the examiners like this approach is the increasing number who ask 'I don't want you to tell me the history, just tell me the main problems.')

2. *A succinct history of the main illness*

   This is the most important part of the history where 90% of the marks are awarded. *Don't take short cuts here*, save them for later. As mentioned before, present a chronic history from the beginning. If the patient is a young infant it is then appropriate to start from the pregnancy.

   Try to make sure you have identified and described fully the *cardinal symptoms*, i.e. the symptoms that you think are most important diagnostically (not necessarily the same as the symptoms the mother volunteers).

In a chronic condition such as asthma, make sure you have covered the periods in between exacerbations, and have committed yourself as to whether the child was 100% normal or still subclinically affected at these times.

When you've finished the chronological part of the history, *try to score extra points* by mentioning at this point and with deliberation the answers to:

a. all the remaining questions for the affected organ system (positives and negatives)
b. all the *'clever questions'* that you can think of aimed at helping with the differential diagnosis (again positives and negatives).

In this way if something in, for example, the family history or the past medical history is relevant it will be mentioned at this point instead of later.

In this way *you should now have covered everything of diagnostic importance in the history*. It is now in your interest to hurry through the next five headings and get on to the physical examination as quickly as possible. But always cover each heading to show that you are systematic.

The five headings are:

*3. General system review*

You have already covered the affected system. Don't waste time on insignificant complaints. Ideally you will be able to say 'There were no significant complaints in the other organ systems'. But remember you have a 5–10% chance of picking up something unexpected, like asthma or nocturnal enuresis, at this stage.

*4. Past medical history*

Again get this out of the way as quickly as possible. If, for example, the case is one of epilepsy, the important details about birth history and previous head injuries and/or meningitis will already have been covered.

It is convenient to include birth and perinatal history, development and immunizations under this heading. Avoid dwelling on any of these in the older child (in whom current school attainments are a far better guide to the future).

*5. Family history*

Do not confuse with social history. This heading really means family *medical* history. Again, important positives and negatives should already have been mentioned.

It is easy to take a history in such a way that one misses the death of a sibling (or a stillbirth) because it is not volunteered. Try to avoid missing such an important event in the life of a family. Again, if one does uncover such a tragedy, it may be appropriate to mention it at the beginning; e.g. 'Susan, who is $4\frac{1}{2}$, is the only surviving child of an unfortunate young couple whose son Mark died in this hospital of leukaemia last year...'

6. *Social history*

    This area is extremely important, as the examiners know it is their only chance to assess your skill and sensitivity at analysing the interaction of medical and social/emotional problems. Even in the case that appears most 'purely organic', there is always the emotional reaction of the family and child to the organic problem, and the social implications in terms, for example, of schooling loss for the child. Try to make definite statements as to the adequacy or otherwise of the family response. If there are major social problems, make sure that you do them justice.

7. *Drug history, allergies*

    (Can be included under past medical history if you like, but don't miss, for example, allergy to penicillin.)

The overriding need in presenting the history is to maintain momentum and not to get stalled on one of the many headings. The danger is that the examiner may waste *your* time chatting about some of his hobby-horses, e.g. tonsillectomy, constipation, teething, etc., if you give him the slightest opening.

*Do not pause* at the end of the history and ask permission to proceed to the examination — go straight on to the examination without even taking a breath.

### On examination

Here again the essential tactic is to present all the positive physical signs, *and all the important negatives* without having to be asked for them. In addition you must *avoid wasting* time (or going down blind alleys) on the normal systems.

Again a comprehensive introduction to this part of the presentation is in order, 'setting the scene', and including the findings on *general inspection.* Include the essential measurements of height, weight (and skull circumference where appropriate) here, giving centiles rather than actual readings and commenting where appropriate on discrepancies. Thus 'On examination I found a boy who looked rather thin for his height, and in fact this was confirmed by finding his weight on the 3rd centile with height on the 25th. There was no gross muscle wasting, no peripheral oedema, jaundice, clubbing or lymphadenopathy but I thought he *was* clinically anaemic. *The cardiovascular, respiratory and central nervous systems were substantially normal (just think how much time you have saved with these ten words!)* the main physical signs being in the alimentary system and these were as follows...'

There are two different ways to present your findings in the affected system. Either:

1. Describe your findings as they were elicited in the usual order e.g. 'on inspection I found... on palpation I found... and on percussion...; I conclude that the patient has a pleural effusion'.

*or*

2. Boldly state your anatomical diagnosis and *then* give the positive physical signs in support of it; e.g. 'the patient appears to have a left pleural effusion of moderate size, *because* at the left base posteriorly there was stony dullness to percussion, diminished vocal fremitus and resonance, with absent breath sounds. There was aegophony at the upper level of dullness. The respiratory movements were correspondingly diminished on the left, and the apex beat was located at the left sternal edge suggesting considerable mediastinal shift.'

Method 1 is reasonably safe but rather cumbersome. Method 2 is preferable and is very impressive when it comes off. It is almost essential for short cases where brevity and polish are at a premium.

Note that both methods are *two-stage* procedures. Never just give your physical signs without drawing a conclusion (some candidates think this is 'playing safe', but they are wrong!) nor give your anatomical diagnosis without justifying it in the same breath.

Be prepared for the examiner to ask you to demonstrate how you elicited the physical signs. Remember to sit down or ideally *kneel* when palpating the abdomen ('Examiners love to see you kneel — Pappworth). Here is the time to demonstrate your rapport with the child and mother. Greet the child by name, flash a smile at Mum to which she will hopefully respond! Talk to the child in a relaxed manner while you examine her — too many candidates because of tension forget even the most elementary courtesies, thus annoying the examiner and increasing their chance of failure.

### Differential diagnosis and management

Whether or not you have to break off to demonstrate physical signs, try at some stage (preferably *before* going to the bedside) to wind up your performance with a crescendo in which you give a nice summary of your findings, leading on to your differential diagnosis. Remember to include social and emotional problems in your summary where appropriate. The whole purpose of the approach outlined above is to give you time for this stage. If you get here uninterrupted and have a good discussion you have almost certainly done well.

### Speed

Think of the long case as being similar to the sport of show-jumping. The rider has to cover the whole course without making any mistakes. The winner is the one who gets round the fastest, with extra marks to be awarded for style.

Don't let the examiner waste your time. If you find yourself getting into an argument about something — stop arguing, concede the point gracefully and continue with your presentation. Similarly, if the examiner points out a relatively minor deficiency in your history (e.g. inadequate details of a hospital admission 10 years ago) don't get all defensive, just *apologise* and get on with it.

*Long versus short cases*

Many candidates who have failed swear that they sailed through the long case and came down in the short cases. This belief is probably exaggerated or mistaken. Examiners say that when they put their heads together they find they have all made roughly the same assessment of the candidate. It is just that the long case *seems* easy, and when the short cases go wrong it is so horribly obvious. If an examiner hears a rather brief and inadequate history, he may keep smiling benignly while secretly failing the candidate. The implication of all this is that one should strive for absolute perfection in the long case. (If you achieve it, it might tip the balance if your performance elsewhere is borderline.)

*Attitude*

The examination is not just a test of factual knowledge and clinical skill. The examiner is looking for all the qualities that make a good doctor and agreeable colleague. Imagine the examiner asking: 'Would I like this person to be the registrar on my ward next week?'

Hence the importance of establishing rapport with your patients, and of *showing* you have done so. Even more important is to **establish rapport with the examiner**. He has to realize you are a nice guy! On entering the room *try* to appear relaxed even if close to vomiting. **Establish and maintain eye contact** with both examiners, giving them both a respectful smile. When asked what seems a fatuous question, avoid showing your feelings, or repeating it back at him with a note of indignation in your voice (surprisingly common). Try to see the best in the question and give a reasonable answer (the odds are it *was* a reasonable question and you just failed to understand the point of it because you weren't on the same wavelength).

**Don't argue with the examiner** — there are no prizes for this whatsoever. Examiners are only human beings, and they have to fail a lot of candidates — it is only natural that they will tend to fail candidates to whom they take a dislike.

Look critically at your own personality and how it affects your exam chances. Perhaps you are a nice, modest, diffident type who wouldn't hurt a fly. If you are, this is fine for life but can be a handicap in the exam! Try consciously to adopt a more extrovert manner, to talk louder and more emphatically. If on the other hand you are naturally on the cocky, self-assertive side, try to tone it down a bit and behave with more modesty and decorum, lest you tempt the examiner to take you down a peg. Whichever the case you are unlikely to overcompensate.

*Keep trying right up to the bell*

Often a candidate despairs and gives up trying halfway through a viva/clinical because he feels he is doing so badly. If you feel like this, take a deep breath, pull yourself together and keep trying. You will be in an emotionally labile state and your judgement is likely to be impaired. Once a candidate gave up so spectacularly in a viva that he ended up being rude to the examiners; he did so because he was convinced he had failed the preceding clinicals. In fact he hadn't, but he failed the viva as a result!

*Miscellaneous points*

1. Avoid using abbreviations (especially in cardiology) — they can be a source of irritation to an examiner.
2. Avoid medical 'slang' for the same reasons, e.g. 'the patient was dripped'.
3. Use proper (pharmacological) drug names, not brand names.
4. Try to detect and eradicate any little mannerisms of speech or behaviour that might annoy the examiner, e.g. saying 'you know' at the end of every sentence, scratching your head frequently, etc.
5. Try at all times to get on the same *wavelength* as the examiner. Try to draw him in to a two-way exchange, and be ready to respond to any cues he gives of encouragement or discouragement. Pappworth says that some vivas are really a game in which the examiner says 'Try to guess the cause I am thinking of'!
   Sometimes the examiner gets so 'drawn in' that he starts teaching you — this is a good thing, as it shows he thinks you worth teaching!
6. Try not to be too clever. There is a tendency to feel that one has to demonstrate extraordinary cleverness to get through this exam. This may, for example, lead the candidate to resort to small-print stuff too soon, looking for non-existent catches in straightforward questions, and most importantly *failing to state the obvious* as if it were beneath him.
   It is far better to regard the exam as more concerned with basics and to talk about common causes before rare ones, answer questions straightforwardly and, above all, to *state the reasons* for your answers at all times to show you are thinking and not just guessing.

*Short case technique*

Short cases are a difficult problem and many candidates feel they are rather an unnatural and unfair way of examining. The main problem is the absence of a history and the need to commit oneself rapidly on physical signs. A further problem is uncertainty as to the rules (e.g. can you talk to the patient at all?) and the examiner's instructions (e.g. he may ask you to look at something but penalize you for not doing something else).
   You should adopt an **active** rather than a **passive** approach to the short cases — attack them, use your initiative, *do more than you were asked to*, and try to answer questions even before they are asked.
   Essentially there are three stages to your performance:

1. describe what you see, i.e. the physical signs;

2. draw your conclusions, i.e. the anatomical diagnosis, and *state* them; then,
3. start a discussion on possible causes *without being asked.*

This approach gives you the initiative and ensures that you say plenty. It is far superior to just saying 'the spleen is enlarged' and handing the initiative back to the examiner. He will just say 'why do you say that?' or 'what is it due to?'

It is often preferable to reverse stages 2 and 1 as mentioned under long case technique, for example, 'I think this patient has a large left pleural effusion because I found ...; possible causes include...'.

It is essential *to do more than you are asked to,* using 'wide-angle lenses' (Pappworth). Often there is an additional clue which helps you to make a diagnosis. For instance in a case of spherocytosis, the examiner may say 'feel this tummy'. If you stick to instructions you will feel the spleen, miss the anaemia and jaundice and never know why you failed!

Thus in every case, perform a *general inspection* before going to the affected system. Thus failure to thrive, clubbing, cyanosis, funny face, retardation, etc. will all be noted and *commented upon* by you.

Similarly, often the examiner says 'Listen to this heart'. *Do not* obey him directly, but pretend he said 'Examine this child's cardiovascular system quickly and efficiently'. Your justification is that you cannot interpret the significance of murmurs without knowing whether the patient is cyanosed, the nature of the pulse and the findings on palpation.

Stick to an organ system approach, (e.g. CVS, RS, AIS) and follow the system of inspection, percussion, palpation and auscultation you were taught as a medical student.

### Approach to the patient (short case)

Do not forget to relate to the child and parent as human beings. Shake hands with the child and ask him his age (which will enable you to make a rough guess as to his growth and development). Give the child clear instructions as to what you want him to do (especially if CNS). If palpating abdomen or joints, ask him first if he is sore at all. You need the patient's cooperation and you need the examiner to see you gaining it.

While eliciting your physical signs, **try giving the examiner a running commentary, drawing your conclusions as you go along**. The advantage of this is you are chalking up points all the time, as well as keeping the examiner interested.

### Diagnosis in short cases

Try to avoid committing yourself 100% to one diagnosis (unless it is obvious, e.g. Down syndrome). This is especially important in a cardiac case, where a systolic murmur should be offered as *probably* A (because of *y* and *z*), but *possibly* B or C (because of *v* and *w*, notwithstanding *x*).

*Other clues in short cases*

Examples of clues in other parts of the body that help diagnosis include:

| | |
|---|---|
| abnormal facies and retardation in a heart case | ?hypercalcaemia |
| thinness, tetracycline teeth in a case of bronchiectasis | cystic fibrôsis |
| anaemia, jaundice in a case of splenomegaly | spherocytosis (or other haemolytic anaemia) |
| parent with neurofibromatosis in a case of café-au-lait spots | von Recklinghausen's disease |
| microcephaly, retardation, cataracts in a case of heart disease | congenital rubella syndrome |
| abnormal facies, anaemia, failure to thrive, etc., etc. | hypercalcaemia plus chronic renal failure |

Too often the candidate sees the clues but doesn't volunteer them, instead waiting for permission from the examiner. Don't wait for permission for anything — do it all straight off — the examiners want you to.

*Cardiac short cases*

As already stated, don't be trapped by 'come and listen to this heart' into auscultating too soon. Make the most out of **inspection** and **palpation**. Make your running commentary audible and *emphatic*, committing yourself to definite statements.

*On inspection* look for and *mention the presence or absence of:* cyanosis, clubbing, dyspnoea, intercostal recession (suggesting a left-to-right shunt), chest deformity, scars and anything else obvious such as growth stunting, abnormal facies, etc.

*On palpation* describe the pulse character, have a quick feel of the femorals if possible, then describe the apex and *state* clearly whether or not you have found evidence of left ventricular hypertrophy. Remember that a displaced apex of normal character may be only a sign of ventricular dilatation rather than hypertrophy, and that a *forceful* apex which is not displaced is perfectly good evidence of hypertrophy (e.g. in aortic stenosis). Similarly state whether or not there is a parasternal heave and *therefore* whether or not you think there is right ventricular hypertrophy (this sounds pedantic but you would be surprised how often candidates describe their findings sounding as if they don't know what the signs of LVH and RVH are).

Then state whether or not you can feel a thrill, and whether or not the pulmonary second sound is accentuated on palpation.

After auscultating, describe your findings, including a *thorough* description of the murmur (systolic/diastolic, site of maximum intensity, timing, character, radiation, etc.) and go on to offer a differential diagnosis *without being asked.*

Discuss the pros and cons of each possible diagnosis again without being asked. If considering a left-to-right shunt, state clearly whether or not you are diagnosing pulmonary hypertension (and why).

N.B. Avoid saying *pan*systolic too lightheartedly — it immediately narrows your possibilities to three (VSD, MI or TI, the last two pretty rare).

If your provisional diagnosis is an atrial septal defect, listen for and mention the presence or absence and significance of a tricuspid diastolic murmur.

If a ? ventricular septal defect, ditto for the mitral diastolic.

### Vivas

Again don't be overawed or try to be over-clever. The examiner knows you have done well enough in theoretical knowledge to pass the written. He now wants to make sure that you don't have any bad gaps, and that you can talk sensibly and clearly about a variety of subjects. If he asks for the causes of something for which there is a list of ten causes, don't say 'There are ten causes of this including 1, 2, 3, 4 . . .' because you will forget half of them and he doesn't really want a list. Instead say 'one of the most important causes of this is 1 . . .' and then milk 1 dry for a bit before passing on to 2.

Avoid dogmatism, and the words 'never' and 'always'. In sociopolitical–ethical areas, e.g. pertussis vaccination, state both sides of the argument before committing yourself. Use the word 'controversial' early on in subjects like this. Be prepared for anything that has recently been in the news and/or medical literature.

Viva technique improves with practice, so pair off with a friend and put each other through it, asking your friend questions *you* have prepared but he hasn't, and vice versa. Be *formal* and unhelpful; don't let each other off the hook too soon.

Another general area which most candidates find difficult is 'out-patient problems' because the candidates do mainly in-patient work, and the examiners do mainly out-patients!

### X-ray reporting

Allow yourself 5 seconds of silence before you start talking. Avoid the medical student approach: 'This is a chest X-ray. It is a P.A. It is of a child. The film is over-penetrated. The bony skeleton is normal', drone, drone . . .

Instead, start by describing the major abnormality. Try to describe it so accurately that someone at the end of a telephone could draw it from your description. Avoid gesticulating with your hands and poking at the film with your fingers (surprisingly common). Avoid criticizing the X-ray; it may be the examiner's favourite.

Avoid using diagnostic terms too early. Say what you see, talking in terms of *zones* (upper, mid and lower) rather than lobes. Use adjectives to describe any opacity, e.g. dense, patchy, etc. When you have finished your description, *volunteer a conclusion*. Again, as in short cases, don't over-commit yourself to any one diagnosis when you don't know the whole clinical picture.

With best wishes to all candidates

Nigel Speight